Bruno Felix-Patrício
Diogo Benchimol de Souza

Principles of histomorphometry

Bruno Felix-Patrício
Diogo Benchimol de Souza

Principles of histomorphometry

and some applications

ScienciaScripts

Imprint

Cover image: www.ingimage.com

This book is a translation from the original published under ISBN 978-620-2-04724-1.

Publisher:
Sciencia Scripts
is a trademark of
Dodo Books Indian Ocean Ltd. and OmniScriptum S.R.L publishing group

120 High Road, East Finchley, London, N2 9ED, United Kingdom
Str. Armeneasca 28/1, office 1, Chisinau MD-2012, Republic of Moldova, Europe
Managing Directors: Ieva Konstantinova, Victoria Ursu
info@omniscriptum.com

Printed at: see last page
ISBN: 978-620-2-72111-0

SUMMARY

ANALYSIS OF WORK PRODUCED IN READING AND TEXTUAL PRODUCTION WORKSHOPS IN PORTUGUESE LANGUAGE AND WRITING CLASSES

Joselene Granja Costa Castro Lima[1]

SUMMARY

This research shows the work done by a vocational high school class at Edvaldo Fernandes State College, which was analyzed after their experiences in cultural artistic presentations, which were planned, prepared and executed by the students throughout 2014. This work was a qualitative, ethnographic study and its data was obtained through reports of experiences produced by the students during their Portuguese language and writing classes. The theoretical framework was based on the authors BAHKITIN, NASCIUTTI, PERKINS and ZIMMERMAN, in order to analyze the relationships between cultural artistic presentations, identity and empowerment. The study was combined with reflection on the discourse of the participants involved in the process, enabling a greater understanding of the limitations of presentations and manifestations in the school unit (as an educational element), since it starts from the context of culture in the school and the meanings attributed by the subjects that give meaning to the teaching-learning process.

Keywords: cultural presentations; experiences; reports.

1 Portuguese Language and Writing teacher at Edvaldo Fernandes State College, with a degree in Vernacular Literature and a master's degree in Educational Sciences.

1 INTRODUCTION

This research was carried out with a group of twenty students from the 4th year of secondary school, in the vocational technical course in Computer Maintenance, which began in 2012 until 2014, at the Edvaldo Fernandes State College, located in a suburb of the city of Salvador-Bahia.

During the Portuguese language and writing classes, the students took part in reading and text production workshops in the school's computer lab, in a learning process involving actions and events from the school's daily life and even outside the school environment, in order to contribute to the textual understanding and practice necessary for a better educational formation. These workshops have given the students more opportunities to create and take part in artistic presentations, cultural events, methodological and technological experiments and practices of an innovative and interdisciplinary nature, with the aim of overcoming problems previously identified in the teaching-learning process.

Through reading and writing workshops, the students were instructed to produce an artistic work that would be presented at various cultural events. In this project, which took place in 2014 and began in the Portuguese Language and Writing classes, the students were instructed to plan and construct an artistic work that would be presented at various cultural events, such as: FLICA (Cachoeira International Literary Festival); the opening of an event at the University's Rectory.

Federal University of Bahia; in the school's annual structuring project: the Sarau de Poesia; and in the traditional event of the Institute of Letters of the Federal University of Bahia.

After the students' artistic presentations, they were asked to produce experience reports. After writing the texts, which contained the students' reflections on their performances at the social artistic events, an analysis of these texts began, with regard to the construction of identity and the empowerment of the subject, in the proposed artistic manifestations.

In addition to reflecting on the participation of public school students in certain social spaces and how this can influence the way they feel within society, this work also needs to understand how cultural artistic presentations influence the way they see themselves within society and their contribution to engagement in the school community, making learning a pleasurable activity.

2. ARTISTIC MANIFESTATIONS IN THE EDUCATIONAL SCOPE

Education is a process of individual and social transformation. The various artistic manifestations, as an educational component, are not simply about acquiring skills, but contribute to the learning of fundamental movement patterns, when related to the modalities and when they offer the student a concrete relationship with the world around them. They therefore play a fundamental role as pedagogical content that privileges the subject's intellectual and bodily culture.

Artistic expression has, in its historical and cultural content, countless possibilities for pedagogical work in any subject, especially Portuguese. It enables students to learn about the history of a people, the world, emotion, imagination and the development of new feelings and movements, while also working on corporeality as a whole, as well as stimulating creativity.

It should be noted that the artistic works are related to their territoriality and customs. And this provides indirect information about the students, the region in which they were brought up, their daily lives, allowing the educator to develop their practice as teaching-learning content.

Therefore, teachers of subjects in general, especially Portuguese Language, should be aware that artistic expressions (be they in the form of dance, music, verse and poetry) bring with them the cultural diversity of peoples, teach the meaning of each movement, rhythm, recital and not just exercise steps and choreography, without paying attention to the cultural heritage contained in these expressions. In this way, teachers will be contributing to respecting cultural diversity and valuing individuals based on their origins.

Therefore, understanding that each school institution is unique, it is of the utmost importance to try to understand how this type of presentation of art has been used for learning from the perspective of its own teachers and students. Because giving a voice to these subjects is the best way to get closer to the meanings they attribute to these manifestations, which could reveal possible limiting factors in the context of school culture.

3. EMPOWERMENT

In a nutshell, PERKINS and ZIMMERMAN (1995) define empowerment as "a construct that links individual strengths and competencies, natural help systems and proactive behavior with policies and social change". It involves the creation of responsible organizations and communities, through a process in which the individuals who make them up gain control over their lives and participate democratically in the daily life of different collective arrangements and critically understand their environment.

The definition of empowerment is close to the notion of autonomy, as it refers to the ability of individuals and groups to decide on issues that concern them, to choose between alternative action plans in multiple spheres - political, economic, cultural, psychological, among others.

Empowerment can therefore be thought of as a teleological aspect of public policies. From an emancipatory perspective, empowerment is the process by which individuals, organizations and communities capture resources that allow them to have a voice, visibility, influence and the capacity for action and decision-making. In this sense, it is equivalent to subjects having the power to critically experience the issues that affect their lives.

Social inequality, therefore, disempowers (FRIEDMANN, 1996), depriving the poor of their right to substantive citizenship rights. Empowerment has become an analytical and empirical category in various fields - administration, economics, public health - including political sociology, as well as a tool with which governments, civil society organizations and development agencies seek to transform the lives of people and communities.

4. IDENTITY

The individual's coexistence in society is driven by the adaptations that are necessary within the various existing social structures. Individual impulses can be developed and shaped by the social environment in which the subject is inserted. In the same way, this same environment has been developed and shaped by individuals and their particularities.

From the point of view of classical sociology, the individual is seen as part of society (a larger unit) and as a product of social determinism. In contemporary sociology, on the other hand, the individual occupies a place that includes both his subjectivity and his constructive and modifying action in the environment in which he is inserted (FRIEDMANN, 1996).

JOHN STUART MILL, in Freedom and Utilitarianism, talking about the limits to society's authority over individuals, brings us important elements about the concept of the individual and society. He establishes a relationship, arguing that "individuality concerns the part of life that basically belongs to the individual", while society is interested in the part that concerns the community.

Psychosociology, which studies the relationships that the individual maintains with the social environment, the social and psychological determinisms that act on these relationships, the way in which these relationships are structured and the effects of these interactions, sees the individual as a social actor, endowed with freedom and position within the social context in which he or she is inserted, a member of a culture and as a psychological subject with his or her own particularities.

In order to understand how the social is constituted and how it acts on its members, psychic structures and social structures must be taken into account, since "(...) the organization of psychic life and the unfolding of individual history are built from a social that pre-exists the subject and contributes to the construction of his values, his models and even his affective life" (NASCIUTTI, 1996).

It can therefore be said that living together in society is a determining factor in the psychological and intellectual formation of individuals, who in turn are molded according to the experiences resulting from the environment in which they act and articulate socially.

5. THE CONSTRUCTION OF THE CRITICAL, POLITICAL AND SOCIAL SUBJECT THROUGH THEIR QUESTIONS DESCRIBED IN THE TEXTUAL PRODUCTION

From the reflective analysis of the reports produced, it can be seen that working with different textual genres in the Portuguese language classroom is of paramount importance for the student's academic, intellectual and critical development. Focusing on the genre of the experience report, it was possible to notice the social development of the students, who perceive, question and criticize, thus assuming their social and political position in which they are inserted; always seeking to understand how the social identity of these subjects is constructed through work with textual genres.

The utterance reflects the specific conditions and purposes of each of these spheres, not only through its (thematic) content and verbal style, i.e. the selection of language resources - lexical, phraseological and grammatical resources - but also, and above all, through its compositional construction.

(BAKHTIN, 2003. p. 277)

The process for constructing the experience report started with the cultural artistic activities expressed in music, poetry and jogral that the students developed in the classroom, observing the rehearsal activities for the presentation at FLICA (Cachoeira International Literary Festival) and at the event at the Rectory of the Federal University of Bahia. They selected songs and a poem that dealt with social, political and racial themes, such as: Que Pais é Esse (Urban Legion), Mulher Brasileira (Benito di Paula), Modinha para Gabriela (Gal Costa), "Me gritaram Negra" (Victória Santa Cruz), which were part of the social sphere of the subjects involved. Through the students' reports, we saw the development of the behavior of these political and reflective subjects, who were inserted in a Portuguese language activity that went beyond the confines of the classroom. The subjects discussed through the artistic manifestos permeate the various issues of the social sphere, so it was necessary to use cognitive skills to discuss the themes and their social development, which took place individually and collectively, occurring procedurally through the various rehearsals. The presentation demanded different means of oral, written and gestural expression from the class, since bodily expression is also a way of dialoguing with the audience, who were the recipients participating in the event. The students involved began to identify with and reflect on their performance, which was going to talk about themselves and the social issues that crossed them in the socio-political sphere through the poem, the jogral and the songs they presented, and represented them socially, as BAKHTIN mentions:

"Language is derived from man's need to express himself, to externalize himself. The essence of language, in one way or another, comes down to the spiritual creativity of the individual."

(BAKHTIN, 2003. p. 289)

The preparation for the writing of the students' experience report was an idea based on the various cultural artistic activities that the students were going to carry out in two locations, the Rectory of and FLICA, in the city of Cachoeira. The artistic and political performance presented by the students to the public sounded like shouts of repudiation of corruption in the country, against racial discrimination and the dictatorship of beauty that praises and characterizes light-skinned individuals with straightened hair, as well as orally expressing the value and beauty of black Brazilian women through music. In this way, the questioning and political nature of the students led to a reflection on the construction of these reflective subjects with different social roles that politically left their mark through their performative choices via oral and gestural expressions and which were reported through the written report, the students were moved by their questioning role that questioned the audience present, In the discussions mediated by the artistic presentation, it was possible to identify factors that show that social, reflexive and political identity is being built up through reflection on political and social knowledge, and knowledge of the world lived through individual experience.

The speaker himself as such is, to a certain degree, a respondent, because he is not the first speaker to break the eternal silence of a silent world, and he presupposes not only the existence of the language system he uses, but also the existence of the previous utterances - emanating from himself or from the other - to which his own utterance is linked by some kind of relationship (it is based on them, it polemicizes with them), purely and simply he already supposes them to be known to the listener. (BAKHTIN, 2003, p. 291)

Another predominant aspect in the students' accounts was the emotion expressed by their gratitude (applause) at the recognition of the valuable teamwork of the students involved, the difficulties of working as a group, planning and projecting the steps in the dance, in the jogral, declaimed poetically by the students or sung through the songs, They also reported on the difficulties encountered in achieving success in the presentations, but the will and determination of the team meant that they overcame the adversities encountered; They also reported that the activities were only possible due to the individual and collective efforts of the student body, which made the group's success possible. Working together was important for the students, and it was noted that the experience gained during the process of constructing the presentations through to their execution was a determining factor in the fulfillment of the activities.

This is why man's individual verbal experience takes shape and evolves under the effect of continuous and permanent interaction with the individual utterances of others. It is an experience that can, to a certain extent, be defined as a process of assimilation, more or less creative, of the other person's words (and not the words of the language).

(BAKHTIN, 2003, p. 313-315)

When talking about experience reports, it is necessary to use the reference of

MARCUSCHI (2008). The author talks about the importance of textuality when he mentions that it takes place in a balanced way between form and content, and not as the observance of syntactic aspects or a set of rules of good form. Based on this information given by the author, we noticed the importance of presenting the genre to the students of the fourth year of the school's Computer Science technical course. As a result of the students' experience of the cultural activities, it was noticeable that their writing became more reflective and descriptive about the importance of the presentations, not just as students, but as questioning subjects integrated into society.

The author's creative consciousness does not derive from a linguistic consciousness (in the broad sense of the word) which is nothing more than a passive phase of creation: the phase in which the material is immanently overcome.

(BAKHTIN, 2003. p. 209)

After the presentations by the students from Edvaldo Fernandes State College, the students were asked to write an experience report, a text relating their reflections on the cultural events. The reports were then handed over for reflective analysis and study. The material from these students was necessary in order to note how artistic and cultural activities can stimulate writing and reflection in this citizen in training. From the reports, they explained the importance of teamwork, applause as a demonstration of recognition of what they have done, and expression, whether verbal or non-verbal.

It is clear that, based on the encouragement and guidance given, the students' participation in cultural events and the writing of the experience report can make them reflect on the act of writing. The text comes to be seen as defined by BEAUGRANDE (1997):

"The text is a communicative event in which linguistic, social and cognitive actions converge." (BEAUGRANDE, 1997 apud; MARCHUSCHI, 2008.p.72)

From the French author's quote, we can see how important social events are in the text, whether oral or written. As far as the research is concerned, the presentations were inspired so that these students from the Edvaldo Fernandes State College could tell us how they happened, what emotion they felt in each cultural presentation, in a detailed and reflective way.

6. STUDENT EXPERIENCE REPORTS

Based on the textual production of the experience reports by the students of Edvaldo Fernandes State College, we can see that the artistic choices represented in the dance, music and poetry question political power, social inequality, racial prejudice and family unrest, and how these issues are directly associated with the students' daily lives. For Bakhtin, the richness and variety of genres of discourse are infinite, because human activity is inexhaustible and each activity includes a repertoire of genres that gradually differentiates and expands as each sphere develops and becomes more complex. Based on the reflections on the specificities described in the reports, it is important to address the construction of this subject, who is affected in social relations, both by the problems that surround him and by his inferences from the artistic presentations.

By choosing the song *"Que Pais é Esse?"* by composer, poet and singer Renato Russo, the class constructed a series of questions generated by the corruption, non-compliance and disrespect for the Brazilian Constitution that comes from the political management of the country, the poverty and contempt of political representatives for the favelas and the hope sung in the lyrics of the song "*in the favelas, in the senate, dirt everywhere, no one respects the constitution, but everyone believes in the future of the nation!*" This choice revealed the students' political vision, based on their autonomy to articulate questions that were expressed through music and body movements in privileged spaces, such as the UFBA Rectory, where one of their performances took place. Mobilizing students to raise political issues outside the school environment and community provides a way of strengthening the student's own awareness of certain social issues.

In the recitation of the poem *"Me Gritaram Negra"* by the author Victória Santa Cruz, , which was also staged by the student body at the Rectory of the Federal University of Bahia, there is recognition of the racial prejudice suffered by the vast majority of the population. The poem points out that after years of fighting racism, the black population has won its place of recognition; and this acceptance is explicit in the poem performed by the class.

In *Genres of Discourse,* BAKHTIN says that "language penetrates life through the concrete enunciations that realize it and it is also through concrete enunciations that life penetrates language". From this perspective, the students also presented *"Mulher Brasileira" (Brazilian Woman*) by Benito di Paula, showing the representation of women in Brazilian society, as well as samba as a cultural and musical activity. They used this opportunity to praise the characteristics of Brazilian women, who in their social circle are mothers, daughters, aunts, nieces, wives and mostly black.

In affirming their identity, the students conclude with "Modinha para Gabriela", by singer Gal Costa. From all these choices, it is possible to see the position of the critical, reflective subject who is politically constituted in the various social spaces.

In an attempt to present the discourse of the subjects who produced the reports, it should be made clear that the students involved in the construction of the experience reports are from the last grade of high school and that the excerpts from their texts reveal the subjectivity produced through the emotions they felt in the rehearsals and presentations, also showing that they have built up knowledge beyond the classroom.

In fragment 1, from an excerpt of an experience report, it can be seen how important the activity was for the student "JOÂO", because according to him:

"It was an activity that made a great contribution to my life, as it dealt with the problem of carrying out group activities and showing them to a large and unknown audience, as well as broadening my knowledge of literature, music and culture" (JOÂO, 2014).

The student's appreciation of literature, music and culture is notable. Moving the student to academic and cultural spaces gives them a perception of new horizons and not just what the physical structure of the school can provide. Through displacement and diverse experiences, the student will be able to develop a critical and reflective perception of the construction of certain social values. In fragment 2, it is possible to discuss and highlight the relevance of the presentations experienced, according to an excerpt from the report by the student "PEDRO", because according to him:

"The experiences I had at the Rectory and FLICA were very constructive. It takes a lot of preparation and dedication for events as important as these. For me, the experience didn't start on the day, it started with every detail. It was more rewarding at the Rectory, because the audience was very captivated by our performance, they reacted with a standing ovation, and that was very motivating. I felt happy to be carrying out this experience, and it will be something that will stay with me forever" (PEDRO, 2014).

The most important thing is that the students interact in a meaningful way and participate in the preparation of the presentations, selecting every detail, work and activity that identifies them and that they like the most so that it can serve as a motivating factor for them.

In fragment 3, it is stated that motivation was an important factor, according to the account of the student "MARCOS", he says that:

"It all started when the teacher told us that we were going to visit the city of Cachoeira and Sâo Felix, but we had to do a performance there, but before we went to FLICA the teacher gave us the proposal to do the performance at the Federal University of Bahia, where we took part in some lectures, events, performances by other groups and then we did our performance where we were very well applauded. A few days after this presentation we went to FLICA, the Cachoeira Literary Fair, where we visited some historic places such as the Casa de Cultura and a cigar factory called Daneman, where a representative showed us the whole process of making and storing cigars. As for the presentation we did, I didn't like it very much because we didn't have an audience when we were presenting, but it was a very good experience" (MARCOS, 2014).

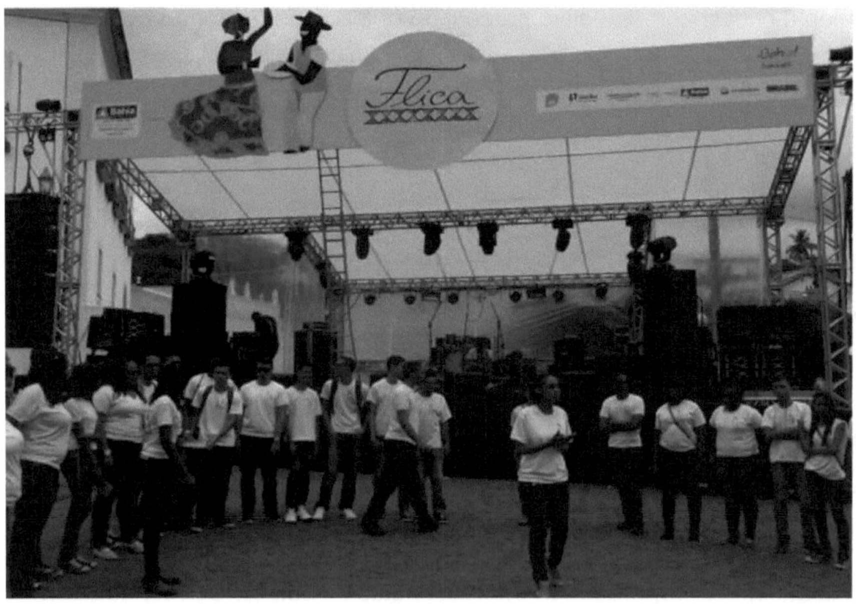

Students presenting artistic manifestations at FLICA (Cachoeira International Literary Festival), in the city of Cachoeira, State of Bahia.

As well as selecting and sorting out evidence of the group's learning, the artistic manifestation made by the technical course class also allowed us to identify issues related to how the students reflect on the real objectives of their role in the group, which of them have been fulfilled and which have not been achieved. In fragment 4, you can see the encouragement in the presentations, as student "ESTELA" says:

"It was something quite different from the presentations at the Rectory because it was the first time I'd been there, so it was intense and I learned a lot and gained experiences that I'll take with me for life, so I'd like to thank the people involved and my colleagues who took part in the presentations with me, and we managed to do a good job after a lot of rehearsals and dedication from everyone. FLICA was easier because we had already been there on another occasion, so we had more confidence because of that experience, but it wasn't any less important for that reason. FLICA is different because it's open to everyone, which makes it even more of a challenge" (ESTELA, 2014).

Working with cultural events encourages students to seek out and intervene in the educational process, from the construction of knowledge to the presentation. In addition to the fact that they feel safe when they are aware of what they are doing and when they are guided to interact with different types of audiences at all times. The important thing is that the mentor teacher invests in building cultural knowledge so that they can become more confident in their presentations, lose their fear of making mistakes and, consequently, learn to develop more.

By taking part in the opening of the event at the Rectory, the students felt safe, realizing that their voices had gained power to express their feelings of justice and social struggle, as they presented problems that are part of their social contexts. In fragment 5, we can see the story of student "ROBERTO":

"The songs presented were chosen by everyone involved in the presentation, they were very good experiences each with their own role in the song, parents and children, I presented the part of the song "I live on the street there's no one" this part my role I went out and lay on the floor as the song says "already lived on the street there's no one, I live in any place, I've lived in so many houses 19 that I don't even remember anymore, I live with my parents". In this excerpt I'll go the way of my respective parents. And in the other presentations we danced, we visited the cigar factory in Cachoeira and other places, we were praised for our presentations and behavior, we were applauded and this may represent that our effort was not in vain" (ROBERTO, 2014).

During the students' presentations, it was possible to observe the support of their families, classmates and teachers. This shows how important support for group work is for obtaining a favorable result in the construction of the individual, both in the educational and social spheres. The participation of parents in one of the events was also of great importance to the project. Although few of them attended their children's performances, they encouraged participation and were always attentive to their children's productions, which made the work much easier. Fragment 6 quotes an excerpt from the report by student "MEIRE", who says:

"For me, the experience didn't start on the day. It started with every detail, the choice of performances, the first rehearsal, you name it."

(MEIRE, 2014).

According to the excerpt above, it can be seen that the subject is built up in social relationships through problem-solving through differences of opinion, as well as by coming together to work as a group during rehearsals.

2014 (the year the reports were made) was the last school year for this class. Admittedly, this way of sharing and becoming aware of learning was new for the participants and for the educators too, despite their habit of reflecting on the necessary practices and interventions. This need to make students aware of what they learn and how they learn involves constant analysis and recognition of the mistakes and successes of everyone involved in the activities.

7. FINAL CONSIDERATION

Reflecting on the reports, it was possible to see that the intervention of this activity gave the students, in addition to the knowledge acquired in the workshop, the opportunity to be present in an academic environment; to produce and present work that was developed with dedication, persistence and excellence, which contributed to a better construction of the identity and empowerment of the high school student who took part in the process. In addition, creativity and teamwork were encouraged, which was also mentioned in the reports analyzed as an enriching experience for the whole class. In view of the results obtained through the reports, it was observed that this meticulous work is gradually succeeding in generating improvements in the quality of public education and helping to form readers who are aware of their political roles in the society in which they are inserted. In this way, students can see the importance of being active citizens, capable of fighting for a fairer and more equal world, with better conditions for the job market.

During the reading of the reports, it was also noted that with each meeting with the class involved, greater integration emerged. Collecting the texts made it possible to discover previously unknown potential. This allowed the students to use their abilities to improve their quality of life. This, of course, has had an impact on their self-esteem, both in their daily lives at school and in their personal development.

It can be seen that any artistic expression makes it possible to look forward to a better life. This could be seen in the discovery of identity and the creative potential of each student, which pointed the way to socialization, leisure, self-knowledge, personal appreciation and autonomy.

Based on the theoretical assumptions and the instruments used in this research work, this study has shown that dance, music and poetry can promote the development of positive change and increase self-esteem, which will contribute to the artistic development of each individual.

8. REFERENCE

BAKTHIN, M. **Aesthetics of verbal creation**. 4.ed., Sâo Paulo: Martins Fontes, 2003.

FRIEDMANN, J. (1996). Empowerment: **an alternative development policy.** Celta: Oeiras.

MARCUSCHI, L. A. **Produçâo textual, análisis de gêneros e compreensâo**. Sâo Paulo: Paràbola Editorial, 2008.

MILL, John Stuart. **Liberty and Utilitarianism**. São Paulo. Editora Martins Fontes, 2000.

NASCIUTTI, Jacyara C. Rochael. **Reflections on the space of Psychosociology**. In: Documenta Eicos, 1996, no. 7.

PERKINS, D.D. (1995). **Speaking truth to power**: empowerment ideology as intervention and policy. American Journal of Community Psychology. Oct. v. 23. n. 5. p. 765-94.

THE TEACHER'S VIEW OF THE PEDAGOGICAL PRACTICES PRODUCED BY PORTUGUESE LANGUAGE AND WRITING WORKSHOPS

Joselene Granja Costa Castro Lima

SUMMARY

The purpose of this paper is to record the actions taken by the Portuguese Language and Writing teacher over the last four years in applying workshops during her lessons in the computer lab room at the Edvaldo Fernandes State School, thus reflecting on the significant results achieved through work developed with the aim of enriching and expanding the learning of students in public primary education, with multimodal reading and textual production practices applied to activities in the area of Language.

Keywords: workshops; practices; production.

1 INTRODUCTION

The first decade of this century has been marked by public policies that have sought to discuss, rethink and reformulate educational processes in Brazil. In this context, education has been providing students with an experience of pedagogical praxis.

The teacher's participation is of fundamental importance in everyday school life and for the work to be successful. They work with the fabric of knowledge, whether from the point of view of teaching, mediating the socialization of knowledge, or as an agent for disseminating what is socially relevant. One of the first activities developed by the Portuguese Language and Writing teacher at the Edvaldo Fernandes State College, located in the city of Salvador - Bahia, was the observation of Portuguese Language classes, with the active participation of the class taking part in the process. This activity was adopted in order to get to know the teaching practice and to adapt it to the school reality. This led to a diagnosis of the needs relating to the didactic-pedagogical perspectives of this subject.

Through classroom observations, the deficiencies related, above all, to the students' textual production were identified. With regard to reading, it was found that the class surveyed had no habit of reading, which could explain the difficulty in understanding text. In addition to these activities at school, we began to analyze and discuss theoretical texts based on the process of textual production and comprehension of the skills of speaking, listening, writing and reading.

The PCN (1997) for Portuguese Language states that "the teaching of Portuguese Language is the expansion of the possibilities of using language, assuming that the abilities to be developed are related to the four basic linguistic skills: speaking, listening, reading and writing".

This work was also based on the reflections of the authors BAKHTIN (2003) and MARCUSCHI (2008), who value textual genres associated with the subject's sociocultural context. According to MARCHUSHI (2008), "textual genres are texts that people encounter in their daily lives, i.e. from experiences in the classroom, with written or spoken enunciations, through interviews, testimonies and so on". According to BAKHTIN (2003) "the various activities of individuals are linked to social practices". For the author, there is also a link between the use of language and the various fields of human activity, as he states in his quote: "all the various fields of human activity are linked to the use of language.

It is perfectly understandable that the character and forms of this use are as multiform as the fields of human activity, which, of course, does not contradict the national unity of a language". This is how the activities were planned for the workshop entitled: "*Portuguese language in the computer lab: teaching reading and producing multimodal texts for technical vocational education*", carried out with classes from the Technical Vocational Course in Computer Science, using technological tools in order to build reflection and practice of digital mechanisms for improving reading and writing, expanding knowledge of some textual genres.

The activity was made a reality by the students' responses when they pointed out their desire to get to know and work with some textual genres, by their textual productions, where informal language and typical internet expressions predominated.

According to the PCN (1997) for Portuguese Language, "the question is not whether to speak right or wrong, but how to speak, taking into account the characteristics of the communication context, i.e. knowing how to adapt the register to the different communicative situations". It is important to emphasize that the teacher's role during the activities of constructing the didactic sequences, which culminated in the workshops, was to guide the textual productions and rewrites of the texts produced by everyone involved in the process.

The construction of the workshops was based on perceptions of some difficulties to be worked on with students in the classroom, leading to a collective construction of meaningful work on some types of textual genres, totaling five workshops applied: on the genres: blog, poster, digital newspaper, charge and the essay workshop for ENEM 2016. As well as allowing students to reflect critically, the practice of doing workshops in the classroom made it possible to develop skills that can be acquired in the teaching-learning process.

2. READING AND TEXTUAL PRODUCTION WORKSHOP FOR THE CREATION OF A BLOG, WITH MULTIMODAL TEXTS

The reading and text production workshops described below were held in the computer room of the Edvaldo State College.

Fernandes, between 2013 and 2016, with the same class, in Portuguese Language and Writing classes.

The activities of producing and understanding text, recognizing the skills of speaking, writing, reading and listening, promote the expansion of the possibilities of using language (BRASIL, PCN, 2000).

Therefore, the first Portuguese language and writing workshop held at the school took place in the school's computer lab, teaching reading and the production of multimodal texts for secondary vocational education, with the creation of blogs whose aim was to use technological tools to help build, together with the school's students, reflection and practice of digital mechanisms to improve reading and writing, expanding knowledge of the textual genre blog. The workshop began in November 2013 and ended in May 2014.

Creation of blogs by the students, as shown below:

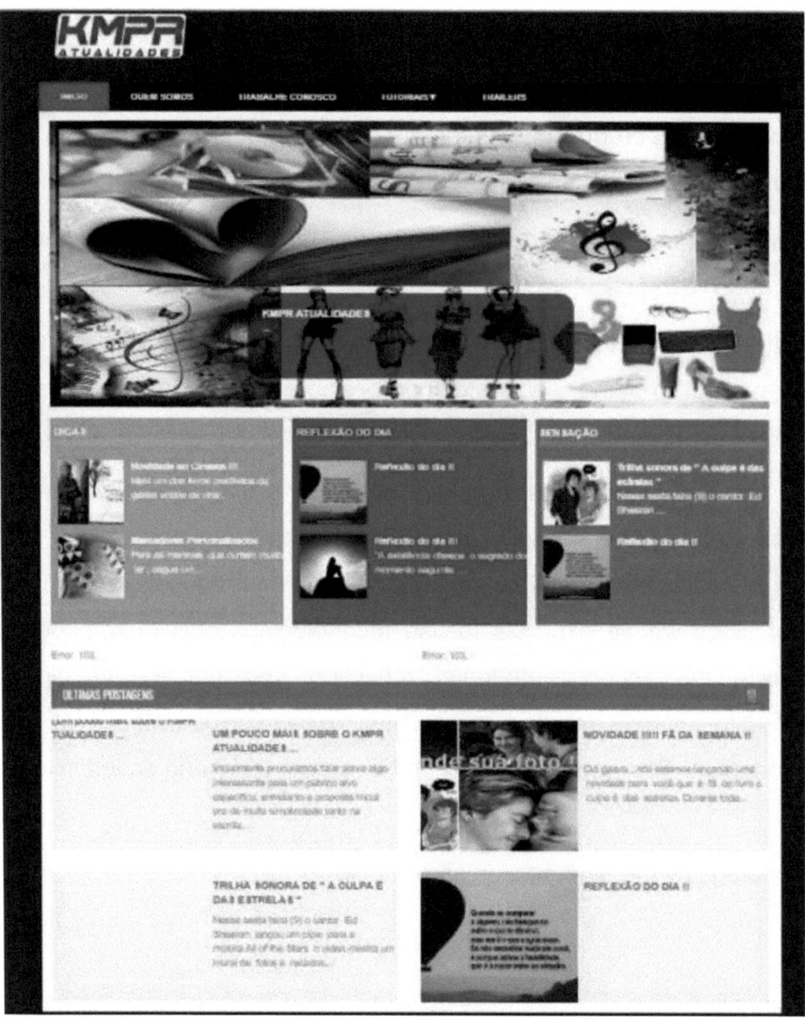

Report by the group that created the KMPR News Blog

Initially, we tried to talk about something interesting for a specific target audience, but the initial proposal was very simple in both the writing and the layout, but always with the idea of creating an electronic magazine. So, little by little, we reformulated the blog, while maintaining the same objective and leaving it with our own profile.

During the vacations, the most frequent posts were daily reflections, fashion updates and previews of the most anticipated and most talked-about movie releases of the moment. As an example, we have posted the trailer for the movie "The Fault in the Stars" and all the other news that has emerged related to this movie, to which we have committed ourselves to posting the news until the movie is released. We know that words can change a person's day, so the daily reflections are a way of telling our readers to live one day after another. To enhance the development of the blog, we now have a tutorials tab where we provide tips and knowledge about CorelDraw, helping you to create your logo and advertisements as well as news about the world of technology. Our blog also contains tutorials teaching some fashion, beauty and health tricks to help people's well-being.

As our aim is to entertain those who visit us, we have also entered into a partnership with the 'RKANIMES' blog, which focuses on making anime available online. Some of the blog's posts have been commented on, which has pushed us to improve every day and satisfy our audience more and more, so we've launched a promotion in which we've selected photos of fans of the book 'The Fault is in the Stars' to highlight as "fan of the week", which will appear on the main slide for seven days.

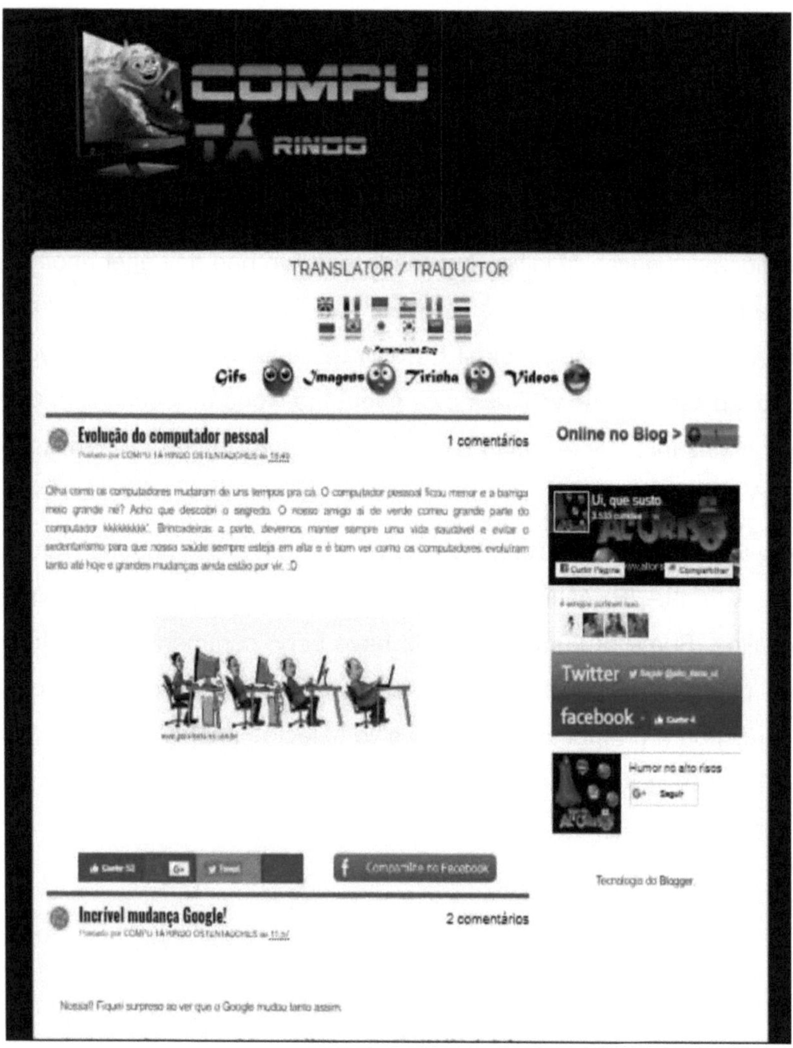

Report by the group that created the Compu tà Rindo blog

We are a group of four computer science students. We've created this blog with the aim of entertaining young people by combining humor with the world of computers.

We hope you enjoy yourselves.

We also have a Facebook profile for people to visit, preferably the girls (kkkk), or those who want to add us and get to know us (kkkkk).

Here we'll be posting humorous content for your entertainment and for those of you who like to have a good laugh. Our aim is to combine technology with humor so that you can have fun and learn at the same time. Is this a way of appealing to you to visit our blog? Of course it is!

VOICE
PÁGINA INICIAL
QUEM SOMOS
DOWNLOADS
FALE CONOSCO
VOICE
VOLTEI!
Feliz Páscoa!
06:30
No comments
Feliz Páscoa
Feliz Páscoa! Que nesta Páscoa haja muitos doces em sua vida. O doce sorriso daqueles que te amam. A doce alegria de ter o pão na sua mesa. A doce esperança de ter um futuro de paz e prosperidade. ...
LER MAIS...
Página inicial
SOCIAL PROFILES
Search
Clique para ativar o plug-in Adobe Flash Player

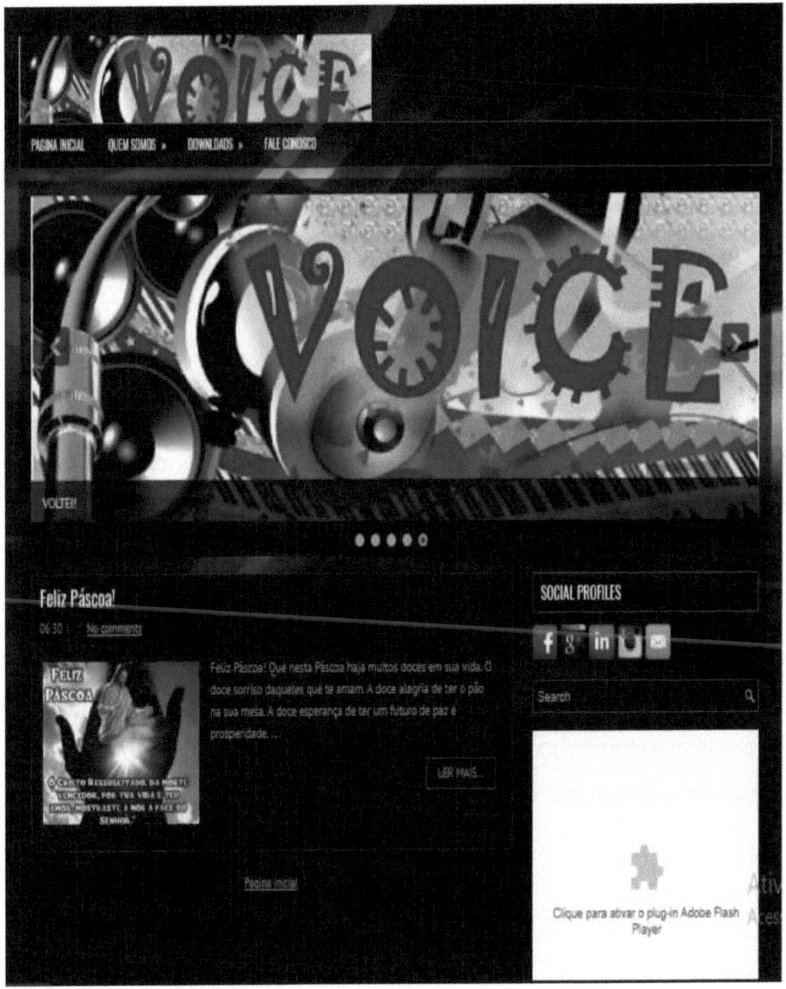

Report by the group that created Blog Voice

When it was suggested that we choose a theme, we opted for something that referred to music and chose the name Voice. Our target audience is music lovers and they can feel free to ask us for any style of music. We're a kind of radio

FM; The public asks for the music they want and we dedicate ourselves to making their choice come true.

In December, our Voice blog underwent changes to its layout, with the aim of improving access for our visitors. With availability of music downloads, the posts have been separated for better appreciation and are also in slide version, which automatically scroll to the top of our blog. We've added a chat feature for communicating with our visitors.

We also cover other subjects on our blog, such as knowledge of the voice, which allows each person to know their vocal type in order to improve their singing and instruments that can accompany the voice according to the accented timbre.

The interest of our Internet users has evolved day by day with new features on the blog that have caught the attention of many people. Today, we've reached such a high level that even people from outside Brazil have gotten to know our blog. The designer has also played an important role in adding new features.

The visitor counter is now located at the bottom of the page on the right and we've opted to leave the mouse pointer layout in the shape of a musical symbol. There is also the "who we are" section, which has been separated into pages to describe each of the components.

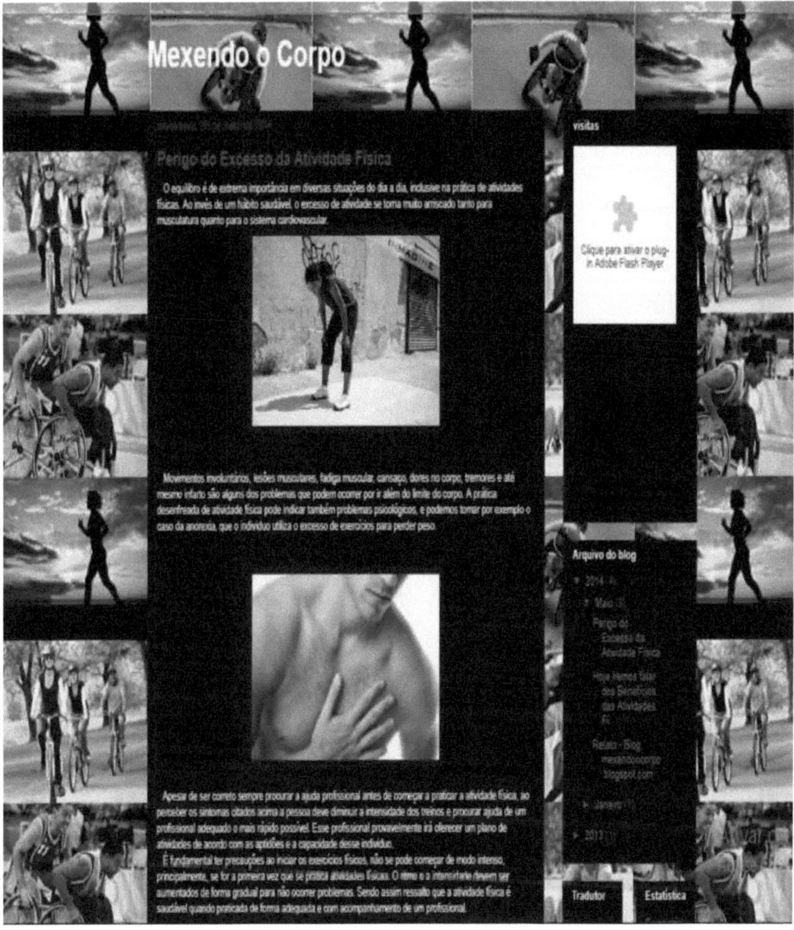

Report by the group that created the Blog Mexendo o Corpo

Based on the team's profile and common interest in physical exercise, we decided to explain the need for and benefits of physical activity.

The initial proposal was to pass on some knowledge of how to take care of the body, what the real need is for exercise, the importance of these practices and the benefits they bring, as well as how to eat properly for a good quality of life.

We have tried to use simple, multimodal language on our blog, using images and text, so that, as well as attracting the reader's attention, it doesn't become monotonous. The proposal is to reach the target audience of young people and teenagers who are interested in maintaining a healthy lifestyle and are not yet aware of the benefits of this practice. However, it is not restricted to young people, as we can often see the growing participation of middle-aged and elderly adults in physical activities to improve their well-being.

It's worth pointing out that even though it's important to exercise, our body is not a machine and needs rest. Physical activity is necessary to stay well and active, even in old age.

Despite seeking instruction in the best and most correct way, it is extremely important that the reader has the support of a qualified professional.

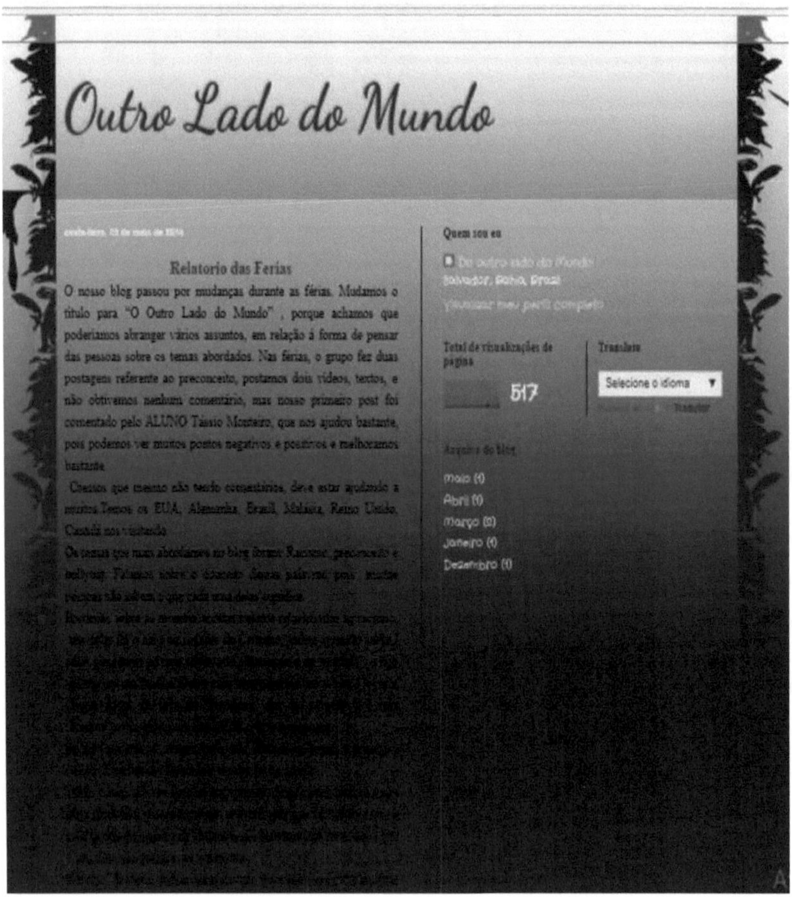

Report by the group that created the blog Another Side of the World

Our blog was created with the aim of addressing issues of racism, prejudice and bullying. We talk about the concept of these words because many people don't know what each of them means. We also talked about recent events in Brazil concerning these issues, one of which was the case of the Cruzeiro player who was verbally attacked by fans of the opposing team who called him a "monkey". Another player to suffer this type of aggression was Daniel Alves, from the Barcelona team, who was hit by a "banana" as he went to take a corner kick. He then made a gesture that no one expected, picked up the banana from the pitch and ate it. This fact has been debated all over the world.

The blog, which even though it's offline and doesn't get many comments, is helping a lot of people because it's being visited by six countries (USA, Germany, Brazil, Malaysia, UK, Canada). So we think they're getting a lot out of it.

3. WORKSHOP ON THE POSTER TEXTUAL GENRE

The second workshop was on the textual genre Poster, the aim of which was to guide the students of the 3rd year of the Computer Technician course at the Edvaldo Fernandes State College in making and producing a collective Poster, using the Google Docs tool, analyzing how this work will be presented at the III World Forum on Professional and Technological Education: Diversity, Citizenship and Innovation, in the city of Recife - Pernambuco. As well as introducing the students to the textual genre Poster, which is widely used in academia, with the aim of providing them with theoretical input so that they can later create and present their own Poster. As well as looking at the choices the students have made for different poster topics, you can show them the topics of a poster (introduction, objective, development, conclusion and bibliography), to familiarize them with the subject matter. After the work presented in class, the poster produced by the students of Edvaldo Fernandes State School will be analyzed and revised. And, finally, to make the student realize that a well-organized and attractive poster, combined with efficient and clear communication, will guarantee an excellent presentation. This workshop began on 13/03/2015 and ran until 17/04/15.

III FÓRUM MUNDIAL DE EDUCAÇÃO PROFISSIONAL E TECNOLÓGICA
Diversidade, Cidadania e Inovação
Assuntos Diversos
PROJETO RÁDIO WEB
Alex Capinam, Ana Paula Belo, Caio Morais, Daniel Sampaio, Danubia Almeida, Dariane, Diana Cristina, Érica Sabrina, Felipe Miranda, Fernando do Carmo, Flavia Dias, Gabriel Luan, Jonathan Anjos, Luan Ramos, Luana Victória, Lucas Santos e Priscila Mourão.
gabriluan@Hotmail.com.;
INTRODUÇÃO
A rádio web é uma transmissão de áudio via internet em tempo real, possível através da tecnologia streaming. Nas rádios web são tocadas músicas ou programações gravadas por locutores. Mas esta última hipótese de áudio não acontece com frequência em uma rádio transmitida online. No caso da nossa rádio web, produzida pelos alunos do 3° ano técnico do Colégio Estadual Edvaldo Fernandes, a transmissão é gravada e são tocadas músicas e programações narradas por locutores.
METODOLOGIA
A radio web é usada como meio de comunicação e entretenimento, funcionando na web, por meio do software gratuito Audacity foi possível editar e mixar o áudio seja ele em wav, aiff, mp3 e ogg e Ustream site responsável por transmitir sons e vídeos através de streaming para o mundo inteiro, os alunos responsáveis se dividiram em setores como: criação de roteiro que envolve notícias, comunicados urgentes e entre outros, locução, criação e organização de playlist e por fim manutenção e manipulação dos equipamentos.
OBJETIVO
O objetivo da web rádio é propiciar maior interação no âmbito escolar, criando um novo ambiente onde toda a comunidade possa de forma interativa pedir música e ouvir notícias sobre temas gerais ou que envolvem a comunidade escolar como comunicados importantes; Toda essa interação expandi o projeto a fim de colocá-lo como um agente social na própria comunidade escolar.
RESULTADOS
Após os esforços dos alunos a rádio web obteve um resultado excelente, mobilizando a comunidade escolar de uma maneira nova explorando uma forma moderna prática e rápida de transmitir notícias e música, fazendo com que o corpo docente e discente da escola aprove o projeto.
CONCLUSÃO
Por fim a implantação da nossa rádio, portanto, foi uma inovação para a nossa comunidade escolar, trazendo informação, entretenimento e tornando-se um sucesso no âmbito escolar. Graças a aprovação e apoio da mesma (docentes, corpo diretivo e principalmente a união dos alunos/ idealizadores do projeto) foi possível melhorar a nossa escola, passando a ser um lugar onde o aprendizado e a produção coletiva sejam os principais focos.
BIBLIOGRAFIA
KOZIEROK. Charles M. The TCP/IP Guide. Disponível em: < http://www.tcpipguide.com/free/t_MessageAddressingandTransmissionMethodsUnicastBroa.htm >. Acesso em 12. 04. 2015.
KARASINSKI. Lucas. Como criar uma rádio online de graça. Disponível em: < ://www.tecmundo.com.br/audio/5454-como-criar-uma-radio-online-de-graca.htm . Acesso em 12. 04. 2015.
ZANELLA. Gislaine. SPRANDEL. Michelle. Perspectivas sobre o conceito de Rádio segundo Mariano Cebrián Herreros. Disponível em: < http://www.intercom.org.br/papers/regionais/sul2009/resumos/R16-0805-1.pdf >. Acesso em: 12. 04. 2015.
BRASIL

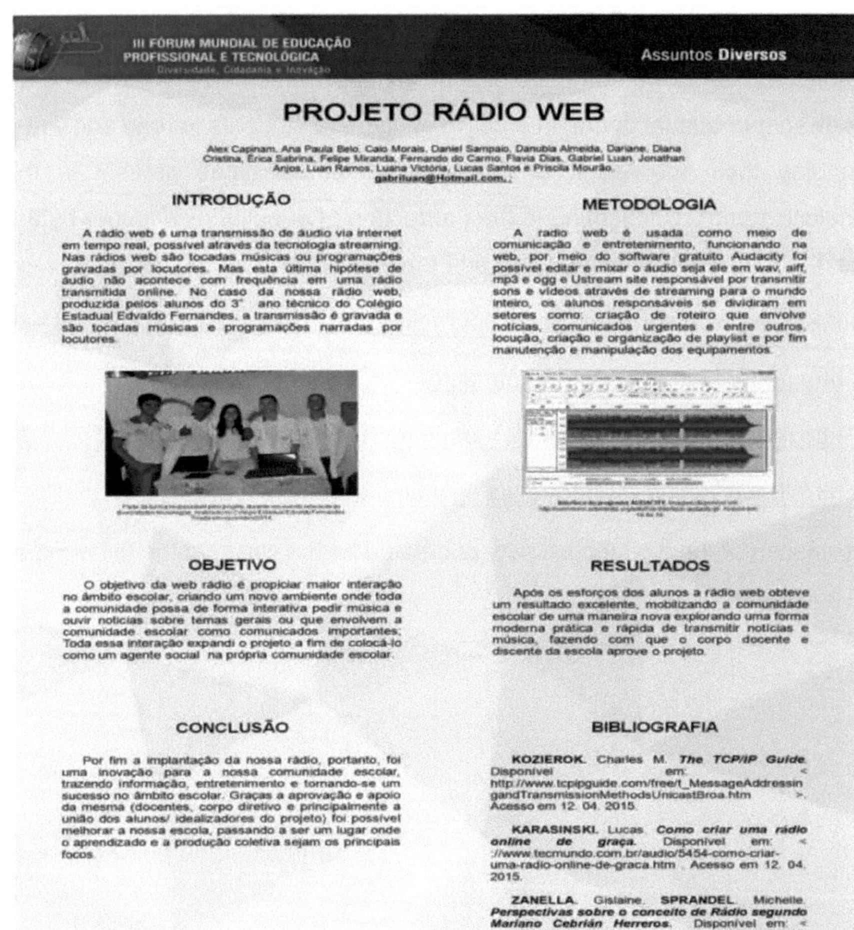

Figure 1: result of the Poster Workshop, created by the class, containing the following aspects: introduction, objective, methodology, results and bibliography.

4. DIGITAL NEWSPAPER PRODUCTION WORKSHOP

The third workshop was on the digital newspaper, with the aim of working on the newspaper textual genre, in order to encourage students to read and write, expanding their knowledge of the different textual types present in the journalistic genre, culminating in the production of a digital newspaper by the class. It began on August 14, 2015 and ran until November 17, 2015.

Results of the workshop on Digital Journaling:

- http://gabriluan.wix.com/iornal-pacto/
- http://teennewsceef. blogspot. com. br/
- http://www.noticiassemfreio.iex.com.br/

Presentation of the digital newspapers created by the class, at the following e-mail addresses:

gabriluan.wixsite.com/jornal-pacto

Crie um site no WIX

"JORNAL O PACTO"

O Jornal da Comunidade

Início Sobre

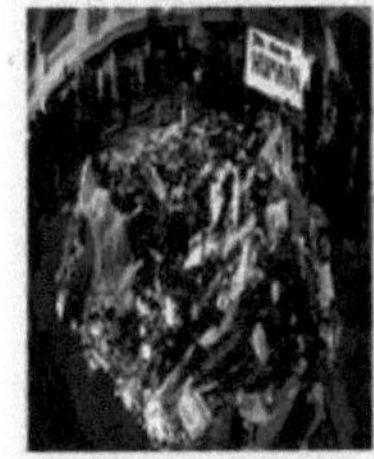

Artigo de Opinião da Semana

28.11.2015

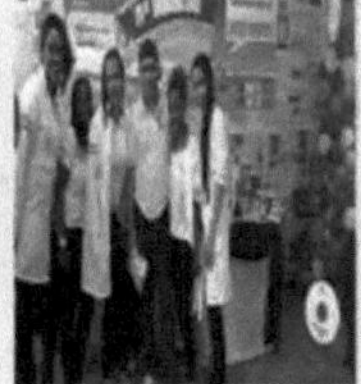

A Feira de Saúde do Edvaldo e o seu objetivo

28.11.2015

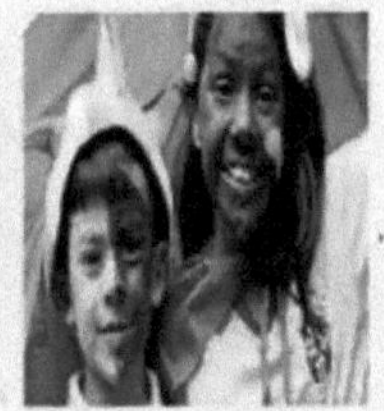

Artigo de Opinião da Semana (Nosso Brasil)

28.11.2015

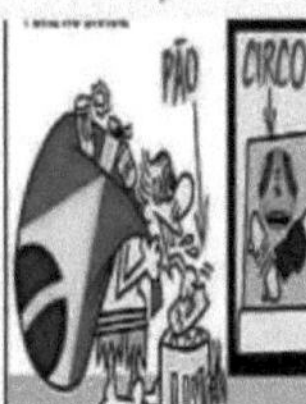

Domingos Redondos (Crônica Especial)

28.11.2015

Artigo de opinião da semana

November 28, 2015 | Luan Ramos

Enviar Notícias

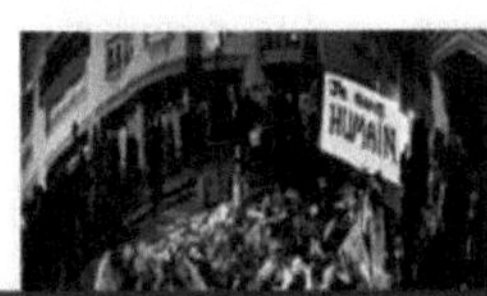

Os dois assuntos mais discutidos hoje em dia estão sendo a barragem que cedeu em Mariana (MG), matando e desabrigando varias pessoas e poluindo o Rio doce, prejudicando toda uma vida marinha que existe nela, e também o ataque sobre a frança que deixaram muitos mortos

Quem somos?

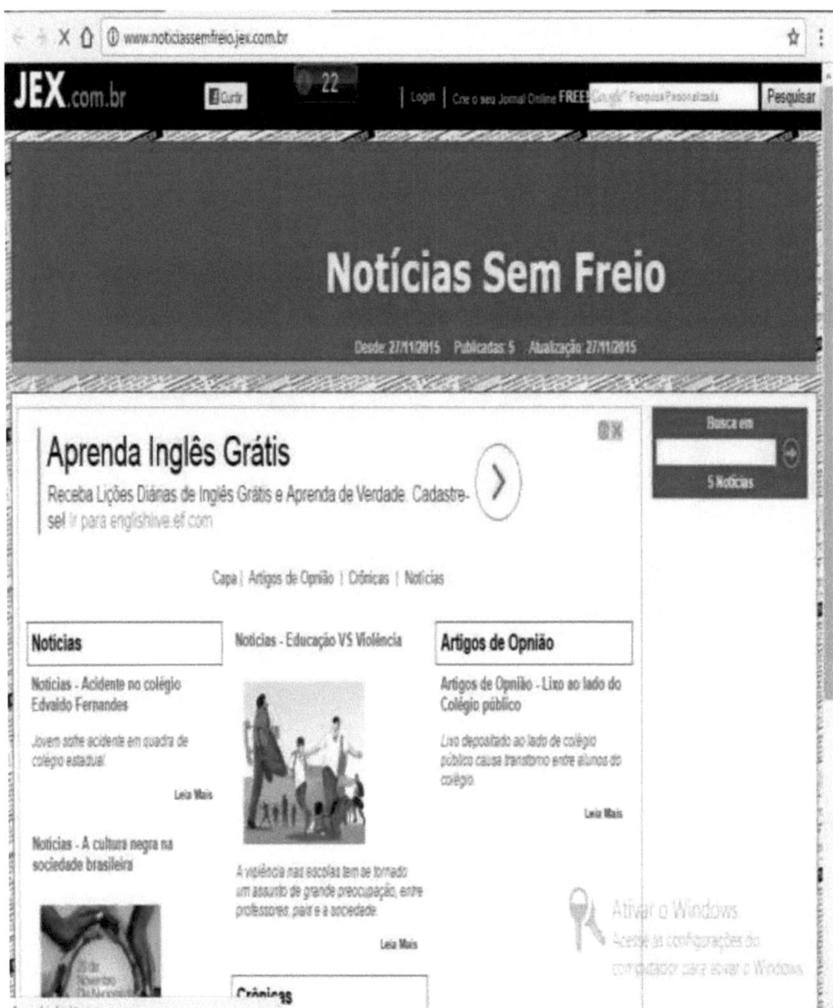
www.noticiassemfreio.jex.com.br
JEX.com.br
Notícias Sem Freio
Aprenda Inglês Grátis
Receba Lições Diárias de Inglês Grátis e Aprenda de Verdade. Cadastre-se!
Capa | Artigos de Opinião | Crônicas | Notícias
Notícias
Notícias - Acidente no colégio Edvaldo Fernandes
Notícias - Educação VS Violência
Artigos de Opinião
Artigos de Opinião - Lixo ao lado do Colégio público
Notícias - A cultura negra na sociedade brasileira
Pesquisar

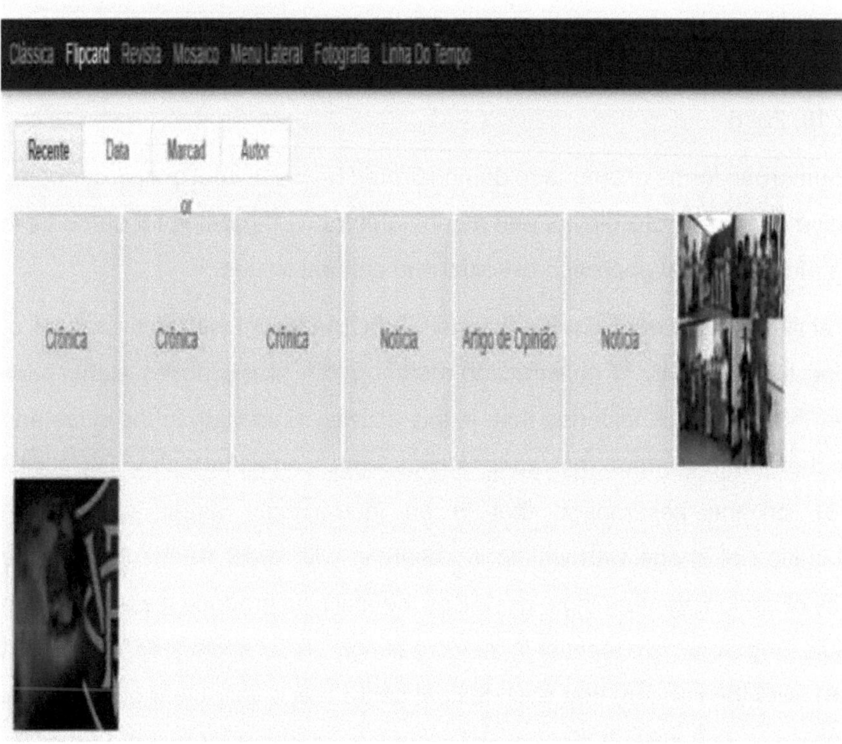
teennewsceef.blogspot.com.br
Teen news O Jornal de todo dia.
pesquisar
Clássica Flipcard Revista Mosaico Menu Lateral Fotografia Linha Do Tempo
Recente Data Marcador Autor
Crônica
Crônica
Crônica
Notícia
Artigo de Opinião
Notícia

5. WORKSHOP ON BUILDING CARTOONS

The fourth workshop was entitled "Constructing Cartoons" and worked with the textual genre in the laboratory during the Portuguese Language and Writing classes. The objective was to carry out a diagnostic investigation, in the form of a questionnaire, of the knowledge about cartoons, applied to the students of the Technical Course in Informatics, which took place on May 6 and ran until June 10, 2016.

The numerous forms of language demonstrated by the textual genre: cartoons, can give rise to a more playful and meaningful form of learning for students in terms of their critical approach to social and cultural issues.

This activity was based on the theorists KOCH (2006), with the concept of reading as an activity of constructing meaning that presupposes author-text-reader interaction, considering that, in this activity, in addition to the clues and signs that the text offers, the reader's knowledge comes into play; DIONISIO (2008), on the assumption that in an increasingly visual society, the combination of image with writing is observed with great frequency and the activity of assigning meanings, as well as the ability to produce messages from multiple languages is essential in an increasingly visual society; MARCUSCHI (2008), with the concept that each textual genre has a very clear purpose that determines it and gives it a sphere of circulation. It has a form and a function, as well as a style and a content, but its determination is basically due to its function and not its form; and BAKHTIN (2003), with the concept that the meaning of a discourse will not only be understood by the words that make it up, but that, in order for it to be fully understood, it is necessary to analyze the whole situation, in which the interlocutors are of paramount importance, since it is their experience of the world that leads them to recognize/construct a certain ideology. These authors provided support for discussing the new concepts of text, reading and comprehension.

With the emergence of computers, new forms of language and literacy have emerged for the habit of reading in the process of forming critical readers, thus having to analyze and understand not only what is written, but also what is implicit in the text. Living in a digital age means perceiving the world through images, icons, symbols, graphics and drawings, making it important to reflect in order to interpret and produce texts.

The construction of the workshop on cartoons began with the weekly preparation of didactic sequences aimed at the study and construction of multimodal texts, which were applied to high school students on the vocational IT course at the Edvaldo Fernandes State College. This reading and textual production work was carried out with the help of various audiovisual resources, such as: videos, online newspapers, power point, tablets, notebooks, teaching and pedagogical materials, ENEM exams from previous years (which had questions with cartoons) and the textbook itself used during the lessons.

Before the activity was carried out, the whole class was given a quiz to find out how much the students knew about this textual genre. Afterwards, the students were asked to search for examples of cartoons on the internet and, based on the results of the previous survey, the workshop was planned and set up. In total, there were 45 five meetings with the class, covering the structural elements that make up the cartoon, as well as the critical and social elements and objectives of this genre. The activities were followed by an exposition of the content through slides (in power point), videos and conversation circles, in the form of debates; always discussing current issues raised by the media.

The cartoon is a textual genre and a multimodal text and for this reason it is very relevant that it be worked on in the classroom, with the aim of introducing and strengthening the concept of image as text, thus providing a subsidy to promote in students the notions of reading, text and language, in order to encourage pleasure in this type of genre. In addition, the aim was for the students to realize the importance of being attentive to the communicative situations of the discursive genre; to identify how dialogue is used in the cartoon; to point out the different types of balloons within the cartoon; to be able to identify the differences between cartoons and comic strips; and finally, to learn how to construct a cartoon using the application indicated later on, or by other means they might wish to research.

At the end of this workshop, the final works created by the four previously divided groups of students were presented, which included the elaboration and construction of a cartoon and a report on the making and production of this activity. In this way, all the students in the class who took part in the process produced, as a team, a cartoon with a free theme and presented it to their classmates. As a result, it was possible to see from the reports written by the students that the workshop had aroused significant interest, not only in terms of producing the work requested, but also in understanding and interpreting the genre discussed throughout the workshop, which helped them to solve questions in the classroom and in exams such as the ENEM and entrance exams they were about to take.

Below are the results achieved in the production of cartoons created by the four teams that were formed to carry out the final work:

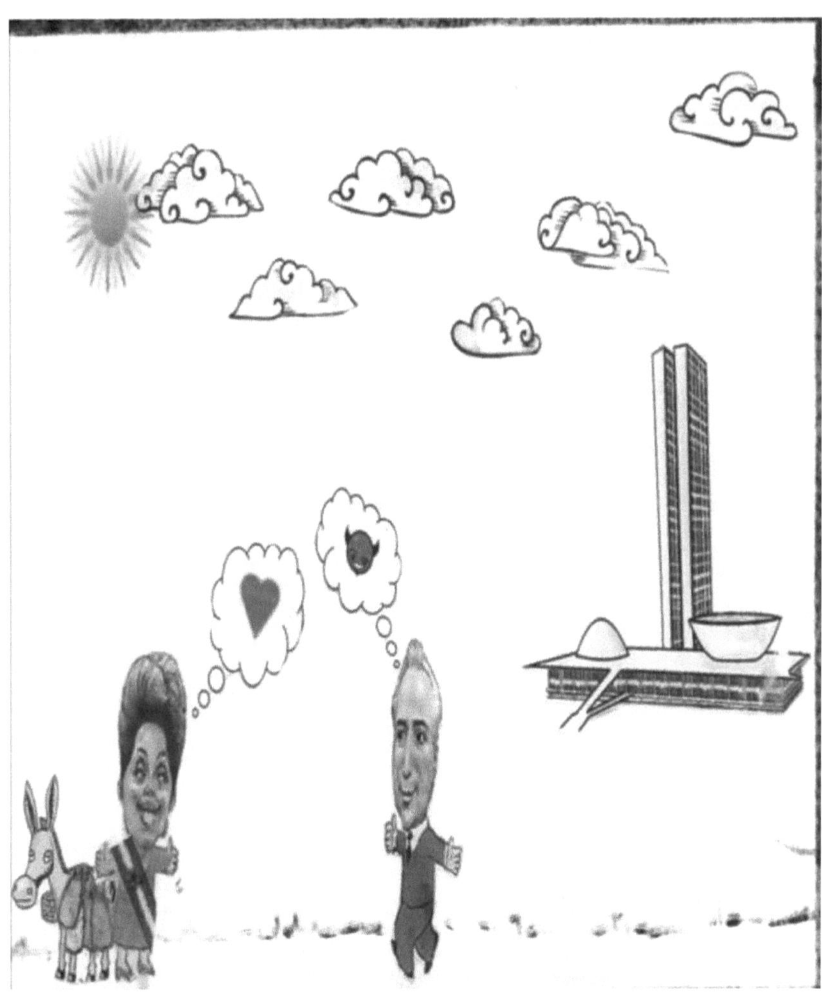

Figure 1: Cartoon about Brazilian politics, where Dilma and Temer show a supposed 'friendship' and the Brazilian people are represented by the animal "donkey". Presented on 10/06/2016

NEWS
JOVEN DE 16 ANOS É ESTUPRADA POR 33 INDIVÍDUOS.
COMO ANDA A IGREJA PADRE?
ESTÁ INDO BEM MEU FILHO. OS FIEIS ESTÃO PAGANDO O DIZIMO EM DIA
BAR SIDADÃOS DE BEM
NEWS
CLARO, ELA ERA AMIGA DOS ACUZADOS.
MERECIDO.
SE ESTIVESSE NA IGREJA, ISSO NÃO TERIA ACONTÉCIDO
PELO VISTO NÃO FORAM SÓ 33 INDIVÍDUOS.
BAR SIDADÃOS DE BEM

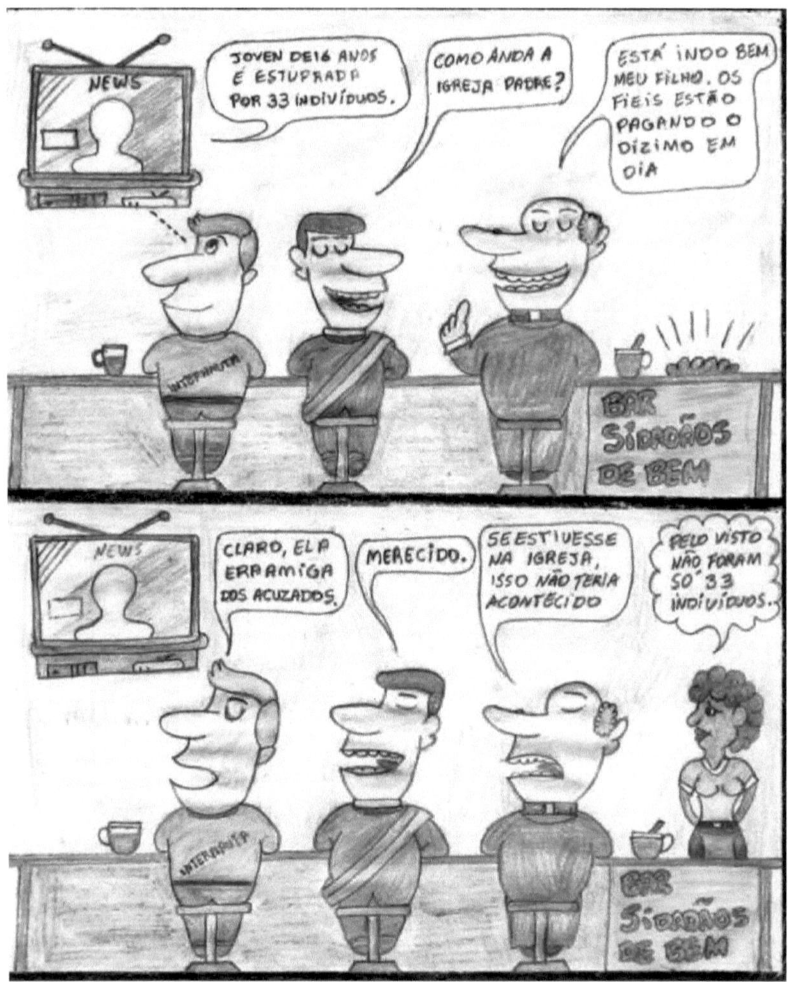

Figure 2: Cartoon about the young woman who was raped by 33 men. Presented on 10/06/2016

COLÉGIOS PÚBLICOS 2016
DIRETOR, PROFES-SOR TECNICO, MERENDEIRAS
AUSENTE!
PROFESSOR de MATEMÁTICA, PORTUGUÊS...
AUSENTE!
ALUNOS...
PRESENTE!

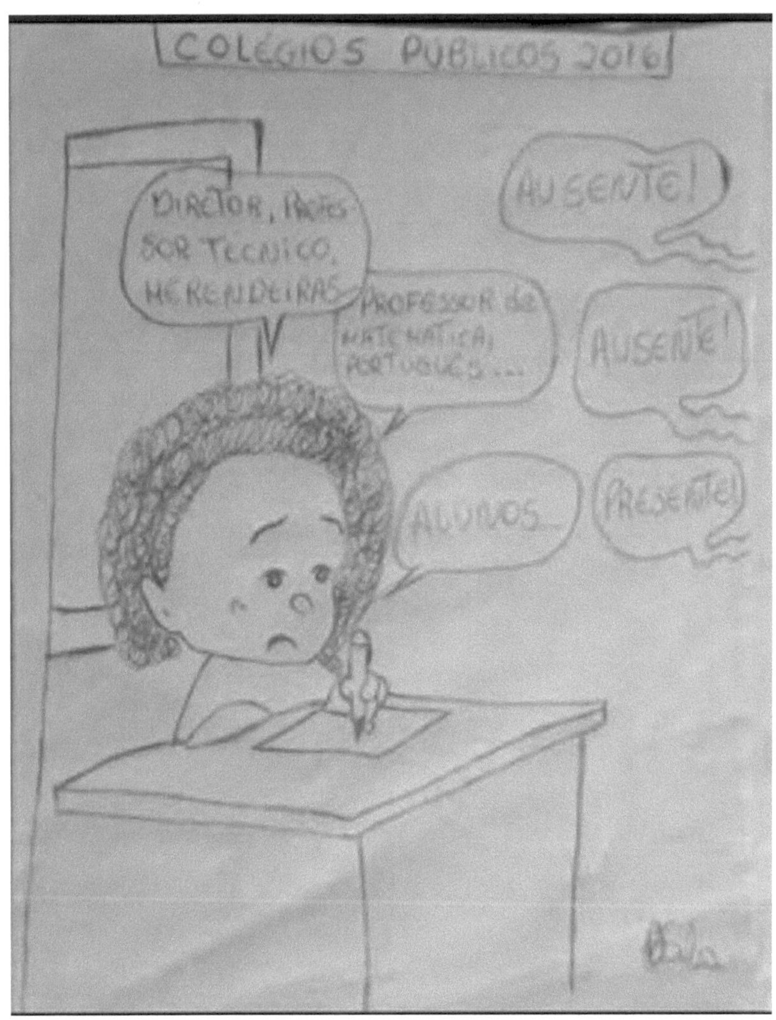

Figura 3: Cartoon about the lack of staff, teachers and teachers themselves in public schools. Presented on 10/06/2016

FILHO! NÃO SAIA SEM COMER, EM 5 MINUTOS O CAFÉ TÁ PRONTO!
COLÉGIO
HAHAHA MÃE EU ESTUDO EM COLÉGIO PÚBLICO EM 2 MINUTOS TO EM CASA!

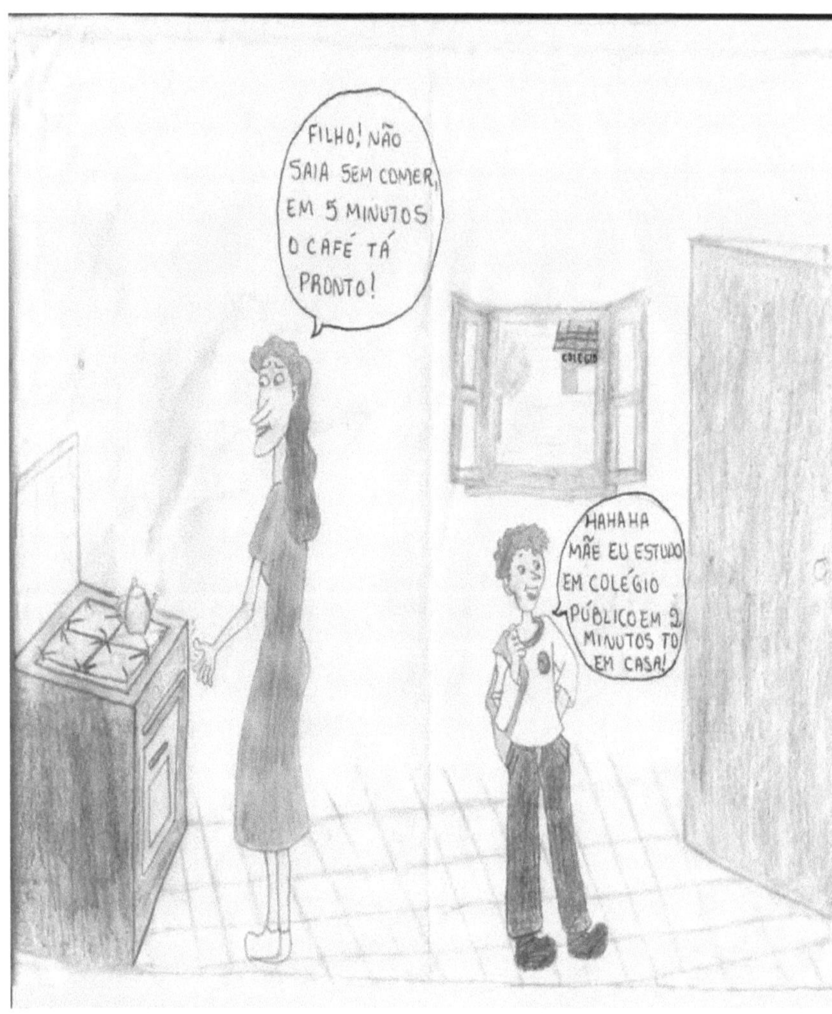

Figura 4: Cartoon about the lack of classes in public schools. Presented on 10/06/2016

6. ESSAY WORKSHOP FOR ENEM PREPARATION

The last workshop given to the class was Writing for ENEM preparation, with the students of the vocational technical course constructing argumentative dissertation texts. The aim was to improve the writing of argumentative dissertative texts (the type of text covered in the National High School Exam), leading students to produce texts that focus on the topic and present a good proposal for intervention.

This activity presents a series of basic concepts for writing an essay, such as mastering the formal written form of the Portuguese language; the correct use of textual typology; the concatenation of the ideas presented to defend a point of view, containing a very diverse socio-cultural repertoire; the construction of a text with many cohesive elements; and the elaboration of an excellent proposal for intervention, without, of course, violating any principle of human rights. However, it is known that it is necessary to have knowledge of the general and specific characteristics for the production of a good dissertative-argumentative text, with a satisfactory structure and a good argument, using criticality in a coherent manner. This will give students the opportunity to learn a little more about writing a text.

The fifth and final workshop was to reinforce the creation of texts for the students taking part in the process so that, by the day of the ENEM, they would have made a significant change to their written productions, applied during the workshop, with the help of didactic sequences developed on a weekly basis. Initially, the components of the type of a dissertative text were presented in class and, based on these, the students began to write their text.

The proposed topic was always discussed first in a conversation circle, so that each student could expand their interpretations and reflections based on the motivating texts, as well as on the discussions at , the opinions of their classmates and the teacher of Writing and Portuguese.

From the very first productions, information was provided that influenced the progress of textual development, such as: using synonyms to avoid repeating words; always paying attention to spelling due to the new spelling agreement; practicing reading to improve writing; and expanding vocabulary, whenever you can keep up with world news and events, and especially in Brazil, which is the aim of the exam topics.

At first, the students were asked to write their essays at home, as they had more time to do so. However, later on, the essays were written in the classroom, under the guidance of the subject teacher, with a set time limit, just like in the national exam.

It is hoped that this work will make it possible to understand the structure that makes up an essay, which is required in ENEM, always using the standard norm to organize ideas, sharpening the critical sense and producing the proposed texts, always keeping the focus on the theme so that the expected competences are successfully achieved.

As authors, we used MARCUSCHI (2008) with his assertion that text is not a product, but a phenomenon, whose existence depends on the processing done by someone in some context, as well as KOCH and ELIAS (2006) with their conception of reading as a meaning-making activity. With the productions made during the workshop, the aim was to create individual portfolios, showing the students' progress and development throughout the learning process.

The results of this workshop were achieved through individual feedback throughout the process, suggesting some improvements on relevant points that were observed during the corrections of the essays written by the students. In this way, the students were able to ask questions about their texts and rewrite them in order to improve their textual productions.

At the end of the work, individual portfolios were produced and given to the students, containing analyses and reflections on the essays, as well as relevant observations to improve and remedy their writing difficulties and, above all, to indicate their progress throughout the process of producing the essays. From the reflections on the texts, it was possible to see significant progress in the students' productions. In many of the texts, the difficulties in writing that were pointed out at the beginning of the workshop were corrected during the process of writing and rewriting the essays.

Finally, there was a relevant observation of the evolution of the teaching-learning progress, according to the reflection of what was scored as inadequate and the feedback given by the students.

7. FINAL CONSIDERATION

The results of the students' participation during the workshops in the Portuguese Language and Writing subjects over the years are substantial, as the students respond positively to the various actions proposed by the project, related to the didactic-pedagogical perspectives of the language area. In addition to demonstrating, with this work, that the moments spent at school have been very enriching, as they bring relevant and remarkable individual and collective experiences to the students.

In this work, it can be seen that despite all the difficulties reported, there is a dedication on the part of the group involved in the learning process, which makes it possible for what is being proposed to go smoothly, in order to improve the use of the students' potential and for them to be helped in the construction of their identity as active citizens and in the transformation of the reality in which they live. The school is a place for learning and development, not only of the content that is taught in the classroom, but it is also a place to learn the most valuable lessons, one of which is to play a very important role in society that is not restricted to learning only in the public space of the school environment.

The opportunity to develop reading and text production workshops, through the creation of didactic sequences, motivating students to actively participate in the school's structuring projects, encouraging the creation of seminars and symposiums, as well as being in direct contact with public school students, is an enriching and healthy teaching experience.

8. REFERENCE

BAKHTIN, M. ***Aesthetics of verbal creation****. 4.* ed. Translated by Paulo Bezerra. Sâo Paulo: Martins Fontes, 2003.

BAKHTIN, M. ***The genres of discourse***. In: BAKHTIN, M. Aesthetics of verbal creation. Sâo Paulo: Martins Fontes, 2003. p.261-306.

BRAZIL, Secretariat for Primary Education. ***National Curriculum Parameters: Portuguese Language***. Brasilia: MEC/SEF, 1997.

DIONISIO, Ângela Paiva. ***Multimodal genres and multilearning.*** In: KARWOSKI, Acir Mârio; GAYDECZKA, Beatriz; BRITO, Karim Siebeneicher (eds). *Textual genres: reflections and teaching*. Rio de Janeiro: Nova Fronteira, 2008, p. 119-132.

KOCH, Ingedore Villaça; ELIAS, Vanda Maria. ***Reading and understanding****: the meanings of the text*. Sâo Paulo: Contexto, 2006

MARCUSCHI, L. A. ***Textual production, genre analysis and comprehension***. Sâo Paulo: Paràbola Editorial, 2008.

A REREADING OF LITERARY TEXTS BASED ON WORKSHOPS HELD IN HIGH SCHOOL CLASSES AT EDVALDO FERNANDES STATE SCHOOL

Joselene Granja Costa Castro Lima[2]

SUMMARY

The aim of this study is to provide opportunities for the development of linguistic competences, as well as to search for and revisit essential foundations, skills and strategies for the reception and production of literary texts with transposition into theatrical language, with a view to the integral formation of the student and based on workshops for this purpose. This work is part of a bibliographical survey, which allowed us to reaffirm the specificity of the biographical fact in socialization processes and to interrogate the field of knowledge open to this research, describing biographical activities, thus seeking individual narratives that cannot be constructed in any other way than on the basis of collaborative research. The conclusion is that it is very important to understand that when analyzing literary works, it is necessary to emphasize what you want to show the students, what you want to provide in terms of knowledge and learning. Thus, the issue of teaching literature or literary reading involves the exercise of recognizing the singularities and properties that nuance a particular type of reading, writing, analysis and construction of meanings.

Keywords: texts; literary; reading.

2 Graduated in Vernacular Literature from the Catholic University of Salvador - UCSAL, teacher of Portuguese Language and Writing at the Edvaldo Fernandes State College, Master's student in Educational Sciences.

1 INTRODUCTION

Adolescence is a period in which people experience important and decisive moments in their psychosocial development which, in addition to the acquisition of a definitive body image, mark the reassessment and incorporation of values, norms and rules which will form part of their adult behavioral repertoire.

It is important for Portuguese language and writing teachers to develop activities, i.e. reading and text production workshops that stimulate reflection in their students so that they can contribute to their growth, bringing literary texts into the classroom, correlated with enjoyable activities that make them participate in the teaching-learning process and become excellent and active readers.

This study proposes a different way of working with reading literary texts in the classroom. It interweaves workshops with dynamic activities that involve and encourage students to rethink their own inappropriate behavior, leading to more fruitful interpersonal relationships.

In addition to instigating the development of values related to the common good, these are important aspects for forming an adolescent identity that is more committed to its own quality of life and that of others with whom it relates, developing social and cultural skills, as well as critical thinking.

When adolescents experience moments of joy, relaxation and mental hygiene, provided by recreational activities such as reading literary texts linked to debates, group dynamics, seminars, dramatizations, among others, the peer group triggers a sense of belonging.

Reading begins with the perceptual process, when we recognize well-known works of literature. Then comes the transfer to intellectual concepts, and the mental task expands from ideas to ever larger units of thought. These mental actions not only consist of understanding the ideas perceived, but also interpreting and evaluating them. These processes are not separated from each other; they merge in the act of reading. There are various ways of stimulating an interest in reading, but often our parents don't know how to read. In this case, we recognize the reasons why the family can't encourage it.

On the other hand, what we do know is that even before learning to read, the child already has knowledge of the world, which we call incidental reading, for example, they don't know how to read the word, but they associate that object with its label, they are already reading even though they haven't mastered the linguistic code.

The aim of this study is to provide an opportunity to develop the linguistic competences, skills and strategies essential for the reception and production of literary texts transposed into theatrical language, with a view to the integral formation of the student.

I'm trying to justify the fact that reading expands oral and written skills, enriching vocabulary and ease of communication and enabling a more solid argumentative base. In addition to theoretical knowledge, it allows us to create, dream, live and relive emotions in a very particular way, without rules or justifications. "Reading good books is training yourself to read life" (RITA FOELKER, 2005).

It is believed that this study is of great relevance, not only to professionals in this field, but to all those who are in some way, even indirectly, connected to this area. Some studies have already been carried out on this subject, but there is little scientific research directly related to this research topic.

It is hoped that this work will contribute information about the practice of reading, taking into account the following problem: How important *is* it for *Portuguese language teachers to develop the use of reading with their students?* This study is based on bibliographical research. The sources include bibliographical research, magazine articles and theses.

2. LEARNING TO READ

Learning to read is a symbolic relationship between what is said and done and what is seen and read. Reading must also be seen as a dual phenomenon involving understanding and comprehension. It is necessary to make a distinction between reading and learning to read. Reading is about establishing communication with texts through the search for understanding.

The activity is an ongoing task that is enriched with new skills as these increasingly complex texts are handled properly. This is why learning to read is not restricted to the first year of school life. It is now known that learning to read is a process that takes place throughout school and throughout life (ZILBERMAN, 1988, p.13).

According to FERREIRO and TEBEROSKY (1991, p. 26), children already have mental constructions about reading and writing before they enter school, and they don't just passively receive knowledge.

According to the authors, the child who arrives at school is already a "good" reader of the world. From a very young age, they begin to observe, anticipate, interpret and interact, giving meaning to the beings, objects and situations around them. They use these same meaning-seeking strategies to understand the literate world.

According to the authors, this natural learning process of reading must be taken into account by teachers and incorporated into their teaching strategies in order to improve the quality of this continuous process, which begins the moment the child is able to grasp and attribute meaning to things in the world. Thus, the action of reading the world in which the child is faced with progressively numerous and varied texts.

The aim of reading at school is to get students to analyze and understand the authors' ideas and to look for the basic elements in the text and the effects of meaning. It is important that the reader gets involved, becomes emotional and acquires a vision of the various message-carrying materials present in the community in which they live (ZILBERMAN, 1988, p.18).

DAUSTER (n.d.), quoted by VAZ et al (1994), redefines the act of reading as the construction of meaning or interpretation by readers with specific skills, identified by positions and dispositions in their reading practice.

Reading takes place when meaning is produced and the more information and previous reading experiences a reader has, the more awareness he or she will have of the formation of meaning, because in addition to what is found in the lines, it is also necessary to look between the lines. Only those who read can interpret, question and make judgments about what they can and should do, fully exercising their citizenship. Only those who read can change reality for the better.

Portuguese is one of the compulsory subjects in the primary and secondary school curriculum. Without knowledge of it, it is impossible for students to understand their surroundings and even to discern the decisions that life imposes on us.

Reading is basically related to the fact that it makes it possible for human beings to succeed, and becoming aware of its importance becomes essential for reading to be highly valued. A good educator values reading and acts consciously by requiring students to read daily at home, going to the library, newspapers, magazines, books, etc.

Reading can't be a mechanical action; on the contrary, it must be demanded, requiring the student to read everything, always encouraging them to take a liking to it.

And to understand it as a whole, you need to learn to read and read a lot. If you do this, you won't find any difficulties in other subjects, because they all depend on reading. The act of reading should accompany human beings throughout their lives. This is very important.

However, school reading is one of the ways of doing reading, because among the students who don't like to read in the classroom are those who use reading in their daily lives, as a sales assistant or reading newspapers, magazines, price lists, etc. The school must provide the conditions for these interactions to take place. In this way, the student advances in the construction of meaningful knowledge through contextualization and interdisciplinarity.

- **AREADING, THE FORMATION OF THE INDIVIDUAL AND SOCIETY**

Reading was once considered simply a means of receiving an important message. Today, the act of reading is a multi-level mental process, which contributes greatly to the development of the intellect. The importance of reading must be recognized by society, because an individual's efficient individual, social and cultural life is based on the habit of reading from the earliest stages of development, because it develops intellectual and spiritual potential, the ability to learn and progress.

Today, children's aptitude for language has declined, while their technical talent has increased. People think that with the advance of technology, the old book no longer has any importance in society. Reading, interpreting, develops critical thinking and reasoning. Without reading, there is no technological progress. Reading means acquiring the ability to explore and understand what you have read. Good reading is a critical confrontation with the text and the author's ideas (BAMBERGER, 1991: 10).

The more we read, the more we are able to interpret a context. Our conception of this read text is a new text. With the relationship between the old text (text read) and the new text (individual interpretation), critical capacity tends to evolve into creative capacity, which generates completely new results.

But it's not just technological developments that have reduced people's aptitude for language. Another factor that undermines the love of reading is the visual stimuli of comic books, as well as all the images broadcast by the media. They restrict the imaginative power of the mind. Reading at an early age should also be considered from the point of view of its influence in counteracting linguistic deformation and impoverishment.

(BAMBERGER, 1991: 11)

This contact with reading must be made before the flood of images in magazines, on television and in comic books takes over the learner, as this will promote their development as a human being.

Readers, during their school years, can only be learners if they don't take a liking to reading. They will never gain autonomy and will miss the opportunity to be transformed by the habit and pleasure that reading provides. The written word is our main tool for understanding the world.

The greatness of the text is that it gives us the chance to reflect on and interpret our society, the world we live in. The book is the starting point for the development of reading. It is therefore urgent, at this point, to take the book in today's education as a continuation of this research.

- **THE ROLE OF READING IN EDUCATION TODAY**

KLEIMAN (1993) explains exactly how reading is approached by teachers and viewed by students. Reading is seen by the student body as something "overwhelming", imposed by the teachers. This is because it is taught the wrong way from the earliest grades.

The school works with textbooks in which the text is just a set of grammatical elements, which are worked on in isolation, out of context, i.e. the message is extracted from the text by understanding and mastering each word one by one.

In fact, the meaning of the text arises from the relationship between its parts, an isolated figure has no meaning, because they are all connected, and this connection is what expresses the general theme of the text.

Another regrettable flaw in reading is to ask questions about the text read, in which the answers are explicitly stated in the text, without any interpretation. As well as making the student practice these tasks mechanically, without using their imagination and reasoning, it is also a disregard for the author, after all, the text is created so that readers can transport themselves into the fiction, often using their own lived experiences. There are specific exercises for working on grammar. There's no need to use a work of art, as this leaves out its real value.

Based on a survey carried out by the aforementioned author, in which she consulted sixty primary school teachers on how they generally approached the text, she unfortunately concluded that they all applied the same script as in the textbooks, i.e. there was no interaction between teacher and student, nor between teacher-text-student.

And it is known from recent research that students don't understand the text when they read it silently, much less when they read it orally. They will understand it when they talk about the relevant aspects of the text, because it clarifies facts that they didn't realize when they read it.

For reading to really take place, the teacher must provide texts with interesting themes for the readers, controversial topics in the press, some subject of interest that arouses their curiosity.

The author also mentions the differences between the written and spoken forms, an important source of difficulty in processing writing, because in speech, there are not as many grammatical demands as in writing, which requires greater elaboration and care in expressions, because in order to understand a written text, it is also necessary to identify, during processing, pronouns and names that are referring to elements that have already been introduced, and which the author does not want to repeat, not least because repetition would overload the working memory.

According to the author: We also do this when we speak, but in writing the distance between the elements that are linked (antecedent and pronoun, repetition or ellipsis) can be much greater (KLEIMAN, 1993, 38).

The poor preparation of texts in textbooks (only isolated excerpts) makes it difficult for students to understand these productions, thus disrupting the process of encouraging reading. Therefore, knowing this deficiency, it is up to the teacher to select only well-written and complete texts to teach students to enjoy reading, and of course, to work with these texts in an interactive way.

According to GERALDI (1984), the basic characteristic of a text is the reader's objective, i.e. the reader must extract information from the text. Knowing how to do this is already a big step towards giving the reader a taste for reading. Reading often becomes torture because the lack of information and imagination is not perceived in the text being read. In schools, for example, there is often no incentive to read.

The teacher tells the student to read a book every week, which will then be worked on in class. After the week, the student returns with the book he has read, but the teacher doesn't work with that text in class. The teacher/mediator should discuss with the pupils, argue the story they have read, because, as has already been said, it is during the conversation between teacher and pupils, in the discussion about the book, that obscure facts that have arisen in the pupil's reading in isolation are clarified.

To answer the question: "What do we do when we read?", Kato (1986) examined the various proposed models of reading, from those that see it solely as an act of decoding sounds to those that see it as an act of identifying the author's intentions and reconstructing the planning of his discourse.

Although the latter comes very close to the behavior and processes of a more mature reader, they consider all these models to be simulations of a particular type of reader's strategy. The mature reader, according to the aforementioned author, acquires the processes cumulatively, and the use of each one is a function of various conditioning factors, such as their maturity, the complexity of the text, the genre, their individual style, etc.

ORLANDI (1988) says that reading, as a proposal to consider it from a discursive perspective, has internal and external objectives. One of the external objectives is to problematize, or rather question, the processes of selecting reading with those who work in its teaching and the internal objective is to learn how "comprehension" works, in the domain of discourse, which means what its mechanisms are, what it represents in terms of discourse, since:

Reflection on the discursive functioning of comprehension has a return that focuses on a crucial issue for discourse analysis itself: the constitution of meaning processes. It's not just those who write that mean; those who read also produce meanings (ORLANDI, 1988).

The author SILVA (1986) explains that the scarcity of reading in the lives of students, and especially teachers, comes from the schooling they have had. She shows us that the educational policy of a certain period sought to impose a school aimed at the "general formation" of all citizens, which prevented any incentive to teach, let alone to read.

The author gives examples of the profile of public schools during this period, justifying the precariousness of teaching which, implicitly, still exists today, with schools that don't have books for their students, and who think that reading is a waste of time, that they would be growing up teaching/learning grammar rules rather than reading and writing texts. This is in contrast to the narrow traditionalist vision of some schools and/or teachers. And, in addition to the few books that schools have, they are extremely precarious in their exploration of reading - which means that there isn't much difference in having these books at school or not.

It is clear that the production of written text is not the main concern of the author of the book, as there were only five proposals for the production of written text in the whole book. This represents more of a challenge to the student's textual competence than an incentive.

The important thing, in this didactic material, is that the student learns the rules of grammar by description, while understanding and producing a text would be a consequence of this practice of learning the language in detail. It was also mentioned that the proposed writing exercises were entitled "text commentaries". In other words, there isn't a single proposal to stimulate and guide the writing process; on the contrary, there are more challenges than incentives for learners.

GONÇALVES (1997), in one of the chapters of his book, discusses the poor preparation of textbooks, in which there are few proposals for the production of written texts. For him, in order to perform well, a teacher must have three theoretical schemes of comprehension:

Draw up a safe and reliable diagnosis of the teaching of your subject, including recognizing the prerequisite learning conditions of your students; making socially relevant objectives explicit; systematizing content that can be fulfilled (GONÇALVES, 1997).

Through these comprehension schemes, we can see that the teacher, when adopting a textbook, should not focus solely on the existing content, but should complement his or her teaching in an attractive and encouraging way for the student, because it has already been seen that what is contained in a textbook (textbook in name only) are only grammar rules, multiple choice exercises or essay questions with an answer induction in the statement itself. What is lacking in textbooks is a didactic approach to writing. In other words, textbooks don't follow the pattern of teaching reading effectively.

We predominantly find in it (textbooks) two extremes that touch each other, identified by their importance: on the one hand, the emphasis on spontaneity and/or "creativity", and on the other, an excess of formal recipes, mainly for dissertations (GONÇALVES, 1997).

3. TEACHING READING AND THE PROCESS OF EFFECTIVE DEVELOPMENT

Reading in the classroom is different from reading a book, a newspaper, a TV program or a magazine in a nonchalant way. Reading in the classroom must advance to deeper levels that allow the student to question, interpret and effectively interrelate with the text. Reading is usually centered on what the teacher wants. He induces the student to read.

Teachers don't guide, they command. When correcting a text produced by their students, they should not place themselves as the judge between the text and the student. But their role should be to mediate in relation to the ideas that have been expressed and in the assessment go beyond correcting grammar.

Textbooks contain, for example, fragments of advertising texts or works by authors and, consequently, there are grammar and interpretation exercises. The question is: how can you interpret a fragment of text? If you don't have the context to at least know the meaning, the message of the text. What about the grammar exercises? You're just asked to remove individual words from the text and then classify them.

The texts, therefore, have no communication with their recipient, they are placed in isolation without context and leave gaps in the student's knowledge. The textbook, for the time being, does not correspond to the creative universe that some teachers seek for their students, because they do not have challenging stimuli for the construction of a personal and cognitive process.

There is an urgent need to rethink the role of the textbook in terms of educational practice and the effective teaching of reading, given the exhaustion of traditional teaching and learning alternatives. Reading has great power, whether literary, formative or informative. These varied readings and languages are the fruit of human knowledge that takes different paths. When we read the world, we must read the various languages that are presented to us, in other words, the various faces of the world.

According to the Parâmetros Curriculares Nacionais - PCN (1997), the formation of readers and, consequently, the formation of writers - people capable of writing effectively, and not, of course, writers in the sense of writing professionals - is due to the practice of reading, because the act of reading gives us the possibility of producing effective texts which, on the one hand, provides us with the raw material for writing: what to write; on the other hand, it contributes to the formation of models: how to write.

Reading should be an object of learning, not just an object of teaching, as it has fundamentally been at school. Reading is not just decoding, converting letters into sound, with comprehension as a consequence, but the school, with this concept of reading, has been training and producing a large number of "readers" capable of decoding any and all texts, but with enormous difficulty in understanding what they read. Reading is interpreting. To interpret is to create meaning, not only from what is written, but also from the knowledge that each reader brings to the text, their knowledge of the world, their life experience.

That's why you can't accept a single interpretation of a text, on the basis that the meaning is given in the text. We need to understand what lies behind the different interpretations, meanings attributed to the same text.

It's up to the teacher and the school to make the student see reading as something interesting and challenging, something that, when conquered piously, gives autonomy and independence. 'A reading practice that does not awaken and cultivate the desire to read is not an efficient pedagogical practice (PCN, 1997, p. 58). An intense reading practice at school is necessary for many reasons, such as broadening readers' world view.

Students often don't have the habit of doing different readings, if they do any at all. As a result, they become narrow-minded in terms of culture. The school therefore has the role of distorting this reality.

It is necessary to reflect with students on the different types of reading and the procedures they require of the reader. These are very different things: reading for fun, reading to write, reading to study, reading to find out what needs to be done, reading to identify the writer's intention, reading to proofread. It's completely different to read in search of meaning - reading in general - and to read in search of inadequacies and errors - reading to proofread. This is a specialized procedure that needs to be taught in all grades, with the degree of depth varying according to the ability of the students.

(PCN, 1997, p. 61)

Another example of the importance of intense reading practice at school is to bring the reader closer to the texts and make them familiar - a prerequisite for fluent reading and text production. This is one of the great shortcomings in training an efficient reader: getting them to enjoy reading. The contact with the text, the proposal to uncover its intention, makes the student understand the communicative function of writing: a text is written to be read.

Reading makes oral, written and other language productions possible; it makes it possible to experience emotions, to exercise fantasy and imagination; it teaches how to study, it makes it possible for the reader to understand the relationship between speech and writing, it expands knowledge about reading itself, it stimulates the desire for other readings, in short, an intense reading practice at school is, above all, necessary, because reading teaches how to read and write.

(PCN, 1997, p. 65)

In short, the reading stirs up our inner selves in a tense and intense way.

It fights with our internal knowledge, poses questions, interjections and reticences that disturb us, making us reflect, interpret, become aware of the depth of a text, thus valuing it.

The next section will describe the goals that were achieved in carrying out this research.

- THE ROLE OF THE PORTUGUESE LANGUAGE TEXTBOOK IN SECONDARY EDUCATION: A LOOK AT LITERARY GENRES

As SOARES (2001) argues, with the democratization of education and the expansion of schools, the concept of the teacher as autonomous and capable of planning and carrying out his or her lessons underwent a transformation, as did the profile of the textbook, which began to explicitly present a teaching methodology with the presence of the teacher's book containing a series of guidelines for teachers and exercises with their respective answers.

Thus, the teacher's autonomy to plan and carry out their lessons is transferred to the material and it imposes itself, assuming the discourse of truth. In this way, as MENDONÇA (2006) states, the textbook presents itself as an opinion-former above the teacher, inserting itself, in the words of FOUCAULT (2006, p. 39), in "[...] societies of discourse, whose function is to preserve or produce discourses, but to make them circulate in a closed space, to distribute them only according to written rules". Therefore, through the textbook and the teachers, the school works towards homogenization.

In addition to developing reading and writing skills, it is the responsibility of Portuguese language teaching, especially at secondary school level, based on literary texts at this level, to promote the practice of analysis and reflection on language. In this context, the textbook at this stage of the schooling process must include a systematized set of works on reading and producing texts which, in addition to integrating literature, also include an approach to textual and literary genres.

When using the textbook in the classroom, one of the interesting aspects of language to be recalled in order to facilitate understanding and demonstrate to students the importance of understanding, interpreting and facilitating communication between educator and student is the linguistic phenomena, textual genres and literary aesthetics that they will work with throughout high school, through language, thus building a relationship with the world in which they are inserted. According to MARQUEZ (1998, p. 34),

Words are memorable, they help us understand how language, in various ways, runs through our existence, giving us humanity, allowing us to look at our past and, through its analysis, transform our present and determine a different future.

It is therefore necessary for students to understand that the study of literature involves reading different texts written by different authors at different times. They must also try to understand the relationship between a particular work and the historical, economic, social and cultural context in which it was produced. The PCN (2001, p. 26) states that:

Thinking about Literature based on this relative autonomy in relation to other ways of apprehending and interpreting reality is to say that we are facing an unusual type of dialogue, governed by games of approach and distance, in which the inventions of language, the establishment of particular points of view, the expression of subjectivity can be mixed with quotations from everyday life, indicative references and even nationalizing procedures. In this sense, by rooting itself in the imagination and constructing new hypotheses and explanatory metaphors, the literary text is another form, a source of knowledge production and apprehension.

However, the main aim of literature lessons should be to turn students into readers of literature. For this to happen, the teacher must first and foremost be a critical reader and be able to stimulate students to read so that they can take a liking to the act of reading.

With this concept in mind, with an understanding of the different forms taken by literary texts and knowledge of the criteria that allow them to be organized into genres, students will be able to see in the text something that transcends a set of words chosen by an author, they will be able to recognize, in that style, the translation of a world view from a personal perspective.

Reading, seen as a sociocultural practice, must be part of a set of social and cultural actions and not exclusively school-based, understood as a practice restricted to the school environment.

Therefore, thinking about reading and textual interpretation goes beyond the scope of the school, but it certainly can't do without it, not least because it is one of the most democratized school institutions that almost everyone can get to and get through, even if, in many cases, some succeed and others do not.

It is clear that the acquisition of reading skills and the study of literature cannot be reduced to presenting a list of authors, works and their dates. Students need to realize that through literary texts they have access to an irreplaceable cultural manifestation. At the same time as the texts give them access to a vision of a historically determined era, the moment in which they were written, they also constitute a particularized manifestation because they translate the vision of their author.

4. FINAL CONSIDERATION

The analysis of secondary school textbooks showed that the use of literary texts was an excellent instrument for the cognitive and social development of students, as well as for the development of basic skills such as reading and writing.

However, these texts, when present in high school textbooks, do not effectively contribute to the construction of students as social and critical subjects, since they limit their proposed activities to mere rereading processes and the "game of search and find", they fail to explore their subjectivity, the construction of meanings and their criticality in a more forceful way, either by allowing them to make their own textual analysis based on the explicit and implicit aspects of the texts, or by making comparisons with other texts and intertextuality, or finally, by presenting their own construction of meanings.

These processes enable these individuals to take a strong stance in the face of different contexts of discursive production, enabling them to deal with the diversity of texts that circulate socially, as well as encouraging the practice of critical and reflective reading of these texts.

In view of the above, it is important to realize that when analyzing literary works, it is necessary to highlight what you want to share with the students, what you want to provide in terms of knowledge and learning.

Thus, the question of teaching literature or literary reading involves the exercise of recognizing the singularities and properties that nuance a particular type of reading, writing, analysis and construction of meanings.

Taken out of context, these procedures contribute little or nothing to the formation of readers capable of recognizing the subtleties, particularities, meanings, depth and relevance to life and social problems of literary constructions.

5. REFERENCE

FOUCAULT, **Michel. The order of discourse**. São Paulo: Loyola, 2006.

GERALDI, Joâo Wanderley. **The text in the classroom 4.** Cascavel: Assoeste, 1984.

GONÇALVES, F. Antenor. **Portuguese Language and Brazilian Literature**. Sâo Paulo: Cortez, 1997.

KATO, Mary A. **No mundo da escrita - uma perspectiva psicolinguistica**. Sâo Paulo: Atica, 1986.

KLEIMAN, Ângela. **Oficina de leitura - teoria e pràtica**. 1. Campinas: UNICAMP, 1993.

MARQUEZ, Gabriel Garcia. **One hundred years of solitude**. 45. ed. Rio de Janeiro: Record, 1998.

MENDONÇA, Marina Célia. **Language and teaching**. Sâo Paulo: Cortez, 2006.

ORLANDI, Eni Pulcinelli. The text: **writing and reading**. Campinas: Pontes, 1988.

SOARES, Magda. **O livro didâtico como fonte para a história da leitura e da formaçâo do professor-leitor**. Campinas (SP): Mercado de letras, 2001.

SILVA, Lilian Lopes Martim. **The schooling of the reader - the didactics of the destruction of reading**. Porto Alegre: Mercado Aberto, 1986.

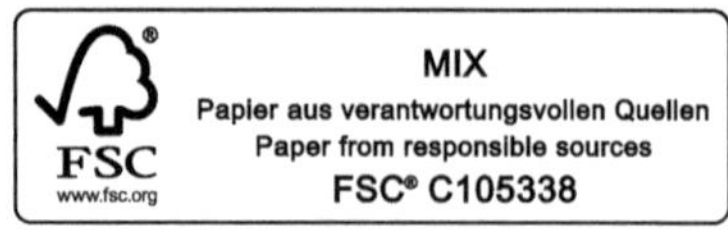

Printed by Books on Demand GmbH, Norderstedt / Germany